IMPLEMENTING EVIDENCE-BASED PRACTICE IN HEALTHCARE

The successful implementation of evidence into practice is dependent on aligning the available evidence to the particular context through the active ingredient of facilitation. Designed to support the widely recognised PARIHS framework, which works as a guide to plan, action and evaluate the implementation of evidence into practice, this book provides a very practical 'how-to' guide for facilitating the whole process.

This text discusses:

- undertaking an initial diagnosis of the context and reaching a consensus on the evidence to be implemented;
- how to link the research evidence with clinical and patients' experience and local information in the form of audit data or patient and staff feedback;
- the range of diagnostic, consensus building and stakeholder consultation methods that can be helpful;
- facilitator roles and facilitation methods, tools and techniques;
- some of the theories that underpin the PARIHS framework and how these have been integrated to inform a revised version of PARIHS.

Including internationally sourced case study examples to illustrate how the facilitation role and facilitation skills have been applied in a range of different healthcare settings, this is the ideal text for those interested in leading or facilitating evidence-based implementation projects, from the planning stage through to evaluation.

Gill Harvey is a Professorial Research Fellow in the School of Nursing, University of Adelaide and Professor of Health Management, Manchester Business School, University of Manchester, UK.

Alison Kitson is Professor and Dean of Nursing, University of Adelaide, Executive Director of Nursing at Central Adelaide Local Health Network (Innovation and Reform) and Associate Fellow, Green Templeton College University of Oxford.

IMPLEMENTING EVIDENCE-BASED PRACTICE IN HEALTHCARE

A facilitation guide

Edited by Gill Harvey and Alison Kitson

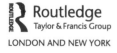

Routledge
Taylor & Francis Group

LONDON AND NEW YORK

First published 2015
by Routledge
2 Park Square, Milton Park, Abingdon, Oxon OX14 4RN

and by Routledge
711 Third Avenue, New York, NY 10017

Routledge is an imprint of the Taylor & Francis Group, an informa business

British Library Cataloguing-in-Publication Data
A catalogue record for this book is available from the British Library

Library of Congress Cataloging-in-Publication Data
Harvey, Gill, 1963- , author.
Implementing evidence-based practice in healthcare : a facilitation
guide/written by Gill Harvey and Alison Kitson.
p. ; cm.
Includes bibliographical references and index.
I. Kitson, Alison L., 1956- , author. II. Title.
[DNLM: 1. Evidence-Based Practice—methods. 2. Health Plan
Implementation—methods. 3. Quality Assurance, Health Care—methods. WB 102.5]
RA425
362.1—dc23
2014039200

ISBN: 978-0-415-82191-9 (hbk)
ISBN: 978-0-415-82192-6 (pbk)
ISBN: 978-0-203-55733-4 (ebk)

Typeset in Bembo
by Swales & Willis Ltd, Exeter, Devon, UK

CONTENTS

CONTRIBUTORS

Ruth Boaden (MA, MSc, PhD) is Director of the National Institute for Health Research (NIHR) Collaboration for Leadership in Applied Health Research and Care (CLAHRC) for Greater Manchester and Professor of Service Operations Management at Manchester Business School (MBS). Her research covers a wide range of health services management issues, with a focus on quality and improvement, as well as the implementation of research into practice. Ruth focuses on knowledge mobilisation arising from high-quality research, ensuring that the findings are accessible and applicable to practice.

Tiffany Conroy (RN, BN, MNSc, FACN, PhD Candidate) is a lecturer and program coordinator for the School of Nursing at the University of Adelaide. Her current role is coordinator of the Bachelor of Nursing (Post Registration) program delivered at the University of Adelaide's Singapore Campus. Tiffany's research interests and publications include the fundamentals of nursing care, knowledge translation, nursing education and the methodology and conduct of systematic reviews. She is completing her PhD investigating 'Factors influencing nurses' delivery of the fundamentals of nursing care'.

Leif Eriksson (RN, MPH, PhD) is a primary healthcare nurse with a PhD in international health. He is post-doctoral researcher at International Maternal and Child Health and junior lecturer at the Department for Public Health and Caring Sciences at Uppsala University, Sweden. His research interests are neonatal health and survival in low- and middle-income countries and knowledge translation.

Vivien Entwistle (RGN) is a practice nurse in Wigan Clinical Commissioning Group (CCG) in England and is also a nurse facilitator for the National Institute for Health Research (NIHR) Collaboration for Leadership in Applied Health Research and Care (CLAHRC) Greater Manchester. She has been involved in all the phases of the GM CLAHRC chronic kidney disease improvement work, in the first collaborative as a practice nurse and in subsequent collaboratives as a facilitator working with colleagues to facilitate and support implementation. She is also a locality nurse 'champion' in Wigan CCG responsible for delivering education across the borough.

Janet Hegarty (MbChB, FRCP) is a consultant in kidney medicine and clinical lead for quality improvement in renal medicine in Salford Royal NHS Foundation Trust. She is also a clinical lead for the National Institute for Health Research (NIHR) Collaboration for Leadership in Applied Health Research and Care (CLAHRC) Greater Manchester, UK. Her experience and interests are in chronic kidney disease, dialysis care, behaviour change and how healthcare services can successfully identify and implement best practice to improve patient experience and outcomes.

Cheryl Holly (EdD, RN, ANEF) is Professor and Associate Dean, Rutgers School of Nursing, Newark, New Jersey, USA and a Fellow in the Academy of Nursing Education. She has an extensive background in teaching, research and quality management, particularly in multi-site partnerships. She has experience in the conduct and teaching of systematic review, particularly meta-analysis, development and evaluation of guidelines, knowledge translation and quality improvement. She holds a joint appointment in the School of Public Health and School of Nursing at Rutgers University, where she teaches systematic review and meta-analysis to nursing, medical and epidemiology students.

John Humphreys (BA, MSc) is a project manager for the National Institute for Health Research (NIHR) Collaboration for Leadership in Applied Health Research and Care (CLAHRC) Greater Manchester. He joined the programme as a facilitator without any clinical background or expertise of project management, instead using the verbal communication skills that he attained from a previous job in the police service to ask lots of questions and learn quickly on the job. The facilitation role has enabled him to build an understanding of what works in practice; to anticipate some common barriers that facilitators and implementing clinicians will encounter; and some experience of how to overcome these issues.

Roman Kislov (MD, MSc, PhD) is a research fellow at Manchester Business School funded by the National Institute for Health Research Collaboration for Leadership in Applied Health Research and Care (NIHR CLAHRC) Greater Manchester. His research focuses on the processes of boundary spanning, facilitation of change and strategy development in large-scale knowledge mobilisation initiatives. Prior to joining academia, he worked as a doctor in a gold mining company in Central Asia, combining clinical work with a senior managerial post.

Katy Rothwell (BSc (Hons), MSc) is currently a programme manager at the National Institute for Health Research (NIHR) Collaboration for Leadership in Applied Health Research and Care (CLAHRC) Greater Manchester, UK, working in close collaboration with NHS, university and third sector partners to deliver a wide range of work programmes including those related to stroke, primary care access and wound care. Her experience and interests cover a wide range of areas including clinical and health service research and evaluation, implementation research and health service management.

Susan Salmond (RN, EdD, ANEF, FAAN) is Professor and Executive Vice Dean of Rutgers University School of Nursing, Newark, New Jersey, USA and serves as the Co-director for the Northeast Center for Evidence Synthesis and Translation. She is a Fellow in the American Academy of Nursing and the Academy of Nursing Education. Her research interests are in the area of urban knowledge translation and systematic review with a special focus in qualitative metasynthesis.

Tim Schultz (BA, BSc(Hons) GradDipl (PublHlth), PhD) is Research Fellow, School of Nursing, University of Adelaide and Technical Director at the Australian Patient Safety Foundation. He is an experienced systematic reviewer and researcher in evidence-based health, focusing on systematic reviews of diagnostic test accuracy and quantitative evaluation of evidence translation activities and patient safety initiatives.

Alison Shanks (BSc, GradDipl (Nutr&Diet), BEd) is Director of Clinical Dietetics at the Royal Adelaide Hospital. Her current role includes a focus on engaging the multi-disciplinary team, including food services, to address malnutrition in hospital. She has facilitated a number of trials and participation in research to support this work. Her broad experience in clinical dietetics, public health nutrition, education and workforce development help her to lead a team of dieticians working in complex clinical care.

Lars Wallin (RN, PhD) is a registered (paediatric) nurse and Professor of Nursing at Dalarna University in Sweden. He is also Director of Research in the regional healthcare organisation – the County Council of Dalarna. Currently he leads a research centre at Dalarna University focusing on implementation and patient safety, where the research programme includes systematic reviews, epidemiological studies, instrument development and trials, all in the field of knowledge translation and implementation research.

Rick Wiechula (RN, BA, BN, MNSc, DNurs) is a registered nurse and senior lecturer and the post-graduate coordinator for the School of Nursing at the University of Adelaide and the Director of the Centre for Evidence-based Practice South Australia, a collaborating centre of the Joanna Briggs Institute. His research interests include knowledge translation, particularly in relation to facilitation of clinicians to improve care. He is also an experienced systematic reviewer conducting orthodox reviews of effect, qualitative systematic reviews and umbrella reviews.

Nancy Whitaker (B.Psych (Hon), M.Psych (Clin)) is a senior psychologist with the South Australian Department of Correctional Services. While working in the University of Adelaide, School of Nursing, she took on the mantle of coordinating the activities of the Centre for Evidence Based Practice, South Australia (CEPSA) a collaborating centre of the Joanna Briggs Institute. Through CEPSA she was involved in a number of facilitation and knowledge translation projects focused on both clinical care and the future of the nursing workforce.

TABLES

FIGURES

PREFACE

This book has evolved from a longstanding involvement in work at the interface between research and practice and a fundamental concern with improving the quality of patient care and healthcare delivery. This has included various programmes of work focusing on quality improvement, practice development, clinical leadership and evidence-based practice. Running throughout these developments has been an interest in facilitation as a mechanism for enabling change and development. When we talk about facilitation we are referring both to roles – facilitators – and a facilitation process that is underpinned by a basic principle of enabling and supporting others to act, as opposed to directing, telling, persuading or coercing.

In 1998, along with a colleague, Brendan McCormack, we published the Promoting Action on Research Implementation in Health Services (PARIHS) framework in an attempt to explain the complex interplay of factors that influenced the implementation of research evidence in the real world context of clinical practice and healthcare. Facilitation was positioned as a core construct of the PARIHS framework, offering a flexible role and process that could anticipate and respond to the complexities of implementation. With a wider group of colleagues - Brendan McCormack, Jo Rycroft-Malone, Kate Seers and Angie Titchen – we continued to develop and refine PARIHS, including testing and evaluating different models of facilitation. The initial idea for this book was to describe a particular model of facilitation that we have used to operationalise PARIHS in our own implementation projects.

During the process of thinking about and writing the book, one of the outcomes has been a re-visiting of the PARIHS framework, because as we systematically reviewed and described facilitation and the facilitator role we had to go back to the original framework and refine the dimensions. The resulting framework that we present in the book is a revision of PARIHS, which we describe as the integrated-PARIHS framework or i-PARIHS. i-PARIHS more clearly positions facilitation as the active ingredient in implementation, working with the core elements of the innovation to be implemented, the recipients of the innovation and the context in which implementation occurs. We outline the details of this and the implications for the facilitator role and the facilitation process as the book unfolds.

However, as a consequence, there are effectively two strands of narrative running throughout the book: one that is telling the story of the PARIHS framework, its history, evolution, development and refinement; the other describing a model of facilitation and its application within the field of implementation practice and research. Obviously the two are connected, but from a reader's perspective, there may be some parts of the book that are of particular interest and relevance. Some may be interested in the earlier chapters of the book where we describe the provenance of the PARIHS framework and the proposed revisions; others may be drawn to the subsequent chapters where we outline the more practical aspects of being a facilitator and facilitating an implementation project. This 'pick and mix' approach to using the book is fine and our expectation is that readers will dip in and out of different sections of the book depending, for example, on whether they are a practitioner or researcher of implementation or where they are in their own facilitation journey. And in the spirit of facilitating learning, we have also prepared some accompanying online resources which aim to help the reader navigate and apply the ideas contained within the book.

Gill Harvey and Alison Kitson

ACKNOWLEDGEMENTS

We have a great many people to acknowledge and thank. First we thank the many colleagues that we have worked with to discuss, deliberate, share and develop the ideas that we present in this book, and in particular, our original PARIHS colleagues – Brendan McCormack, Jo Rycroft-Malone, Kate Seers and Angie Titchen. A special thank you also goes to the many international colleagues we have collaborated with to develop, test and further refine our ideas about facilitation and implementing evidence-based innovation in practice. We also have to acknowledge the numerous healthcare practitioners, patients and managers that we have engaged with along the way checking out the realities of implementation and really finding out what works and what does not. The learning we have gained from these experiences is the foundation for the ideas we present in the book.

1

INTRODUCTION AND OVERVIEW OF THE BOOK

Gill Harvey and Alison Kitson

Why a book on facilitation?

What should we do about the perceived gap between what research suggests is 'best practice' and what actually happens in the real world? How can we speed up the process by which innovations are adopted in healthcare? Which strategies should be used, when and how in order to implement improvements in patient care? These are all frequently heard questions within a healthcare environment, whether talking to policy-makers, managers, clinicians or educators. And the answer is very often a contingent one – 'well, it depends . . . '. But what does it depend upon – and more importantly, what can we do about it?

In this book we draw upon our own and others' experiences of working in the fields of implementation and evidence-based healthcare to try to answer some of these difficult and complex questions. In particular, we set out to describe a practical model of facilitation that can be used to plan, conduct and evaluate real-time implementation projects. We purposefully focus on facilitation as this is a strategy that we have found most helpful to enable and support implementation, because it is interactive, iterative and adaptable – the very opposite of the 'one-size-fits-all' models that claim to offer a magic solution to the problem of implementation. The challenge of implementation is something of a dilemma: there is no proven recipe to follow, yet simply acknowledging that it is complex and challenging is of little help to those charged with a responsibility for implementation. Recognition that the process is messy and difficult may well chime with our lived experience; however, what is needed in practice is some guidance and practical pointers about what to look out for, how to respond and how to move forward in roughly the right direction. In other words, the equivalent of a road map that documents the coordinates, the potential obstacles and the contours to anticipate, but still allows the navigator to plan and agree the exact route to take between points A, B and C. This is our intended objective for this book: to provide the equivalent of a map and compass that will enable facilitators to tackle the tricky terrain of implementing evidence within a real-world setting.

We start off the chapter by outlining what we mean by facilitation and why we believe it is an approach that is well suited to the implementation challenge. In addressing this latter point, we position facilitation within the wider context of developments in evidence-based healthcare and specifically within a framework that we developed over 15 years ago to explain the processes of successfully implementing evidence into practice – the Promoting Action on Research Implementation in Health Services framework, or PARIHS as it is commonly known. PARIHS was developed as a conceptual framework, which suggested that successful implementation was a function of the complex interplay between the evidence to be implemented, the context of implementation and the way in which the implementation process was facilitated. Since its original publication in 1998, the PARIHS framework has been widely used and cited within the field of healthcare. However, this has been mostly as a heuristic to think about implementation at a general level or to retrospectively evaluate why a particular implementation project failed or succeeded. At the same time, questions have been posed about how to use PARIHS in a more prospective way to plan and conduct implementation projects. This requires thinking about how best to operationalise a conceptual framework – something we have been doing in our own practice as facilitators and researchers of implementation. This book documents our learning about the process of facilitation and, through reflecting on this learning process, represents our attempt to operationalise PARIHS by providing a practical guide to the facilitation process and the facilitator role in implementation.

Defining facilitation

Taken literally, the word facilitation means 'to make easier'. It derives from European languages such as the French word *faciliter* and the Italian *facilitare*, which can be traced back to the fourteenth and fifteenth centuries. In everyday use, facilitation is an idea that began to emerge in a variety of disciplines from the mid 1900s onwards, particularly within the so-called 'helping professions', such as education, healthcare and social work, but also more generally in the discipline of management, for example, in relation to leadership and quality improvement. A number of reasons for this have been identified, including the need for more human communication to make sense of an increasingly complex and fast-moving world, with a resulting requirement for greater adaptability, responsiveness and power sharing (Hogan, 2002). Core themes apparent in the emergence of the facilitation concept include participation, engagement, shared power and decision-making. Thus, in education there was a shift from the language of teaching to student-centred and experiential learning, heavily influenced by the humanist psychology of Carl Rogers (Rogers, 1969). In the field of management, the human relations movement had a similar influence in terms of challenging the prevailing views of managers and employees, particularly in terms of promoting greater involvement of employees in decision-making and problem-solving at work (Mayo, 1933). Facilitation was concerned with enabling individuals and groups to reflect upon and understand what they needed to do to change aspects of their work, behaviour, attitudes or relationships with others in order to address problems or achieve specific goals.

This thinking, in turn, influenced approaches to quality management, through the work of theorists such as Deming (Deming, 2000) and Juran (Juran and Godfrey, 1998), emphasising the importance of workers taking responsibility for quality and solving quality-related problems, rather than being subject to inspection and assessment by managers. Other parallel developments include the emergence of co-counselling approaches (Heron, 1989), the growth of participatory research methods such as action research (Reason and Rowan, 1981) and the wider spread and influence of emancipatory approaches in general. Present in all of these developments is a focus (implicit or explicit) on enabling others, rather than telling, directing, persuading or coercing people into action. This emphasis on enabling, helping and making easier is reflected in dictionary definitions of facilitation and the facilitator role (see Box 1.1) and typically involves using processes of experiential learning to support reflection and problem-solving in practice.

BOX 1.1 DEFINITIONS OF FACILITATION

- *Facilitate*: To make (an action, process, etc.) easy or easier; to promote, help forward; to assist in bringing about (a particular end or result).
- *Facilitation*: A means of enabling or promoting; a help, boost, impetus towards attaining a particular goal or result.
- *Facilitator*: A person or organisation assigned to facilitate progress towards a specific objective, especially one whose role is to foster communication or understanding within a group of people, or negotiations between various parties; a mediator; a coordinator.

Source: Oxford English Dictionary; www.oed.com.

At one level, the potential contribution of facilitation to the field of evidence-based healthcare is obvious – it should offer a way of helping to ease the translation of research evidence into practice. But why have we particularly focused on facilitation as a strategy for implementation? And how can this fairly general concept of 'enabling' or 'making easier' be made relevant and practical at the point of implementation? In exploring these questions we will first look briefly at the history and development of both the evidence-based movement and facilitation approaches in healthcare, before explaining how and why we think facilitation has a useful contribution to make to the field.

A brief history of evidence-based healthcare

The founding father of the evidence-based healthcare movement is acknowledged as Archie Cochrane, an epidemiologist and respiratory physician, who having accepted an invitation from the Nuffield Provincial Hospitals' Trust in London, wrote a small book on the lack of scientific evidence upon which to base medical decisions (Cochrane, 1973). Speaking from several years' experience as both a clinician and a researcher, Cochrane outlined his views on how medicine could become more effective by systematically testing how much a medical activity (or any other therapeutic intervention) can change the natural course of a disease. The way this was done was through randomised controlled trials (RCTs) – the gold standard of proving what worked – and from this evidence medical practitioners could begin to discard practices that were ineffective and embrace those that had the evidence to support them.

Cochrane also described the importance of health systems being efficient (utilising their human and capital resources wisely) as well as addressing fundamental values such as equality, access, unnecessary variation and cost. It was not until the early 1990s that these ideas began to filter into more mainstream thinking. In Oxford, England, Iain Chalmers had already begun to develop these ideas in the perinatal epidemiology unit, producing one of the first handbooks on undertaking systematic reviews of evidence of effect (Chalmers and Altman, 1995). The Oxford group, led by Sackett, developed the first Master's Degree in Evidence-Based

Healthcare at the University of Oxford, UK (Dawes et al., 1999). At McMaster University in Canada, the Evidence-Based Medicine Working Group, led by pioneering clinicians such as Gordon Guyatt and David Sackett, similarly challenged the way that clinical decisions were routinely made, suggesting that they were too often based on intuition, unsystematic clinical judgement and peer influence, rather than on robust scientific evidence (Evidence-based Medicine Working Group, 1992; Sackett et al., 1996). To address these concerns, the concept of evidence-based medicine was proposed, whereby physicians were expected to apply skills in literature searching and critical appraisal of scientific papers to inform decisions about patient care. Problem-based learning methods were used to help equip trainee doctors with the skills needed to practice in an evidence-based way.

The ideas and methods of evidence-based practice soon began to permeate into other areas of healthcare, including clinical fields such as nursing and allied health and subsequently into management and policy-making, for example (Lomas, 2000; Walshe and Rundall, 2001; DiCenso et al., 2004). Influenced by the early thinking of the evidence-based medicine movement, initial developments focused largely on making evidence more easily accessible and understandable, for example, through synthesising research evidence in the form of systematic reviews and clinical guidelines and teaching skills in literature searching and critical appraisal. The basic premise was that if research evidence was made more readily available to clinicians, managers and policy-makers and they had the necessary skills to find and interpret the evidence, then they would apply that evidence in their decision-making about patient care or health service planning and delivery. This view of evidence-based practice represents a rational and mostly linear process of decision-making; the assumption being that when 'good' evidence is available, individuals will use it as a matter of course, providing they have the necessary skills and knowledge to do so.

However, despite considerable investment in infrastructure to synthesise research evidence (for example, national and international health technology assessment and clinical guideline development programmes), the work of international groups such as the Cochrane Collaboration and the establishment of educational programmes to develop critical appraisal skills, gaps between research evidence and what happens in practice have persisted (Grol, 2001). Critics have challenged the notion that evidence can simply be transferred from researchers to practitioners (whether at a clinical, managerial or policy level) to be used in an unquestioning and straightforward way. Studies of evidence use in practice illustrate that far from being a logical process, it is typically complex, messy and unpredictable (Dopson and Fitzgerald, 2005). When making decisions about patient care or the organisation and delivery of health services, decision-makers are usually considering research evidence alongside a whole host of other knowledge sources, such as local priorities, resource availability, political saliency, patient needs and preferences, policy and regulatory requirements. Thus research evidence is frequently contested and negotiated and the extent to which it is useful and used depends upon how well it 'fits' into the particular setting (Ferlie et al., 2000). This reinforces findings from studies in the wider field of innovation and management, which demonstrate that a combination of factors influence whether and how new ideas are adopted and implemented, including characteristics of the innovation, characteristics of the adopters, readiness of the system or environment for change and the implementation processes used (Rogers, 1995; Greenhalgh et al., 2004).

As the complexities of implementation were identified, a shift in thinking around evidence-based practice and what it involved also took place. Instead of seeing it as a researcher-led activity of knowledge transfer, the emphasis moved to thinking about it in a non-linear way where researchers and users of evidence both had key roles to play, ideally in a collaborative relationship (Van de Ven and Johnson, 2006). Consequently, the importance of multi-faceted and multi-disciplinary approaches began to be recognised and the language shifted from 'knowledge transfer' to more active and interactive terminology, such as knowledge translation and knowledge mobilisation. Some commentators challenged the very notion of evidence-based decision-making, suggesting that the most that was reasonable to expect – given the contingent nature of evidence and the multiple factors that could influence its uptake – was evidence-aware or evidence-informed policy and practice (Davies et al., 2008).

Running through the debates and discussion about evidence and evidence-based healthcare, a number of common themes are apparent. First, is the view that evidence is broader than research and that 'good' research is not sufficient to guarantee its uptake; second, a recognition that 'context' matters and that factors both within the inner and outer context (i.e. the immediate site of implementation and the wider organisation and policy environment) play a significant role in determining the outcomes of implementation; third, a need to tailor implementation methods and approaches to match the particular needs of the situation. It was within this space that the development of the PARIHS framework was undertaken. Having experienced first hand the challenges involved in implementing clinical guidelines and quality improvement initiatives in healthcare, our lived experience reinforced the complex and multi-faceted nature of implementation. With this widening view of evidence-based healthcare, a range of social science theories have been applied to inform our understanding of implementation. We will introduce and explain a number of these different theories as we move through the book.

A brief history of facilitation in healthcare

In healthcare, the application of facilitation approaches and methods is evident in a range of fields, such as health promotion and primary care prevention programmes, quality improvement and audit, practice development, action research, clinical supervision and knowledge translation, to name just a few. This reflects the broad purpose of facilitation as essentially an enabling or helping process. Early references to facilitation focus on health promotion and particularly the development and implementation of the 'Oxford Model' of preventive health (Fullard et al., 1984). This model was established in the early 1980s to introduce more systematic approaches to coronary heart disease prevention, through identifying and training facilitators who could work with primary healthcare practices to support the establishment of systems such as health checks and routine screening for high-risk patients. The facilitators were external to the practice team and worked with several practices at the same time, providing advice, support and networking opportunities to help the practices introduce new systems and ways of working.

This approach to facilitating health prevention has had a significant influence in the field of primary care, particularly in relation to chronic disease management. Examples of similar facilitated methods of primary care prevention are evident in Europe (Engels et al., 2006), Canada (Liddy et al., 2013), North America (Nutting et al., 2010; Parchman et al., 2013) and Australia (Cockburn et al., 1992) and have been the subject of evaluation studies to determine their impact on health outcomes and processes. For example, a recent systematic review of 23 studies evaluating practice facilitation within primary care settings found that primary care practices were almost three times more likely to adopt evidence-based clinical guidelines when they received facilitator support (Baskerville et al., 2012). In the studies reviewed, the facilitators employed a number of key methods within the overall facilitation intervention, most notably: audit and feedback, interactive consensus building and goal setting, reminder systems, tailoring their approach to the local context and practice needs, use of common quality improvement tools (such as Plan–Do–Study–Act cycles) and system and organisational level change. The first two of these (audit and feedback; interactive consensus building and goal setting) were the most commonly used strategies, adopted in 100% and 91% of the reviewed studies, respectively.

In the field of quality improvement, facilitators have been employed in problem-solving approaches such as quality circles (Ingle and Ingle, 1983) and more recently in quality improvement collaborative approaches, such as the Institute for Healthcare Improvement's breakthrough collaborative model (Institute for Healthcare Improvement, 2003). Here the facilitator plays a central role coordinating and supporting the improvement programme, through facilitating learning events, supporting the local implementation of Plan–Do–Study–Act (PDSA) cycles and maintaining regular contact with participating teams and organisations to monitor progress, assist with problems, maintain motivation and momentum and enable networking. As we will describe in Chapter 2, in our own work in the field of quality improvement (prior to the development of the PARIHS framework), we applied the concept of facilitation as a method for supporting locally based standards and audit systems, which emphasised the importance of teamwork, consensus decision-making and local ownership of quality (Royal College of Nursing, 1990; Morrell and Harvey, 1999).

Another area that has emphasised facilitation and the facilitator role is nursing practice development. In line with models of clinical supervision that emphasise reflective practice and experiential learning (Palmer et al., 1994), the practice development literature is characterised by a central focus on critical reflection, experiential learning and changing practice cultures (see, for example, McCormack et al., 2013). The facilitator's role, therefore, is to enable the process of reflective learning, with a particular emphasis on developing insights that can enable individuals and teams to transform themselves and factors within their organisational environment that may act as barriers to the implementation of change and improvement.

Comparing these examples of facilitation, it is apparent that facilitation – and the corresponding facilitator role – can be interpreted rather differently in practice, from a role that is largely focused on supporting the achievement of a specific objective (or set of goals) to one that is more focused on enabling the transformation of individuals, teams and health systems. This is something that we will explore further as we describe our approach to operationalising facilitation within the PARIHS framework.

Facilitation and evidence-based healthcare

A whole range of roles and methods are described in the literature on knowledge translation that could be broadly categorised as 'facilitation', in that they are concerned with helping to achieve the implementation of evidence into practice. These include, for example, roles such as educational outreach, academic detailing and opinion leaders and methods such as audit and feedback, tailored messaging and education and computerised reminder systems (see, for example, Grimshaw et al., 2012). Indeed the study reported by Baskerville et al. (2012) demonstrated that facilitators commonly used a combination of such methods. We will examine these different roles in some more detail in Chapter 5; but what do we mean when we talk about facilitation and facilitators within the PARIHS framework?

In PARIHS, we identified three core elements that appeared to influence the trajectory of implementation efforts: evidence, context and facilitation. We will explain the PARIHS framework and its constituent elements in more detail in Chapter 2; suffice it to say here that PARIHS positioned facilitation as the active element in the implementation process. In other words, facilitation strategies and facilitator roles were presented as enablers of implementation, offering tailoring mechanisms that could respond to the characteristics of the evidence to be implemented and the particular contextual conditions of the implementation setting. However, as a conceptual framework, PARIHS did not give detailed guidance about how to facilitate. As a PARIHS team we developed and experimented with various approaches to facilitation – some goal-focused and others that were more emancipatory. Indeed, these different perspectives on facilitation were influential in the development of the PARIHS framework, as we will discuss in more detail in the following chapter. In relation to the focus of this book – implementing evidence-based healthcare – our intention is to describe a goal-focused approach to facilitation. This starts from the perspective that there is a desire or need to implement something new, whether that is a clinical guideline, a particular piece of evidence or a service improvement. From this starting point, we will illustrate the range of things that need to be considered within the implementation process to maximise the chances of success, from the characteristics of the 'thing' to be implemented, to the individuals and teams that are targeted during implementation, the setting in which they work and the wider organisation and health system environment. Our intention is to build a map that can help facilitators to plan, guide and evaluate their implementation journey.

An overview of the book

In the chapters that follow we will start to build up our model or map of facilitation, including a discussion of the facilitator role and the skills and knowledge needed to be an effective facilitator. Chapter 2 provides some more information about how and where we started our own facilitation journey: the history of the PARIHS framework and why we developed a central interest in facilitation. In Chapter 3, we will look at our own and others' experiences of applying PARIHS and how PARIHS compares to other implementation models and frameworks that have been developed to inform and guide evidence-based practice in healthcare. We will also consider some of the theoretical literature on innovation, improvement and facilitation and how we think this aligns to the PARIHS view of implementation. Bringing together this theoretical and empirical literature, we will outline our thinking for a revised version of PARIHS, which we describe as the integrated PARIHS or i-PARIHS framework. Chapter 4 builds on the description of the i-PARIHS framework and presents the model of facilitation that we are proposing to activate or operationalise the framework. In Chapter 5, we focus more specifically on the facilitator role – what sort of people make good facilitators, what skills and knowledge they need and the developmental journey from a novice to a more experienced and expert facilitator role. Chapter 6 then starts to illustrate the model of facilitation in action, explaining how facilitation and the facilitator role functions within a specific implementation project, with particular attention to the evidence or innovation being implemented and how the facilitator works with the individuals and teams involved, including taking account of their local context. At this level, we are focusing on the types of implementation activities someone relatively new to the facilitator role might be undertaking, while under the guidance of a more experienced facilitator.

In Chapter 7, we move on to thinking about the facilitation process beyond the immediate life of a project, both in terms of sustaining change once it has been implemented and spreading the initiative to different areas. This involves thinking both about wider contextual issues and the development of more advanced facilitator roles and skills. Having described and illustrated our facilitation model and the roles of novice, experienced and expert facilitators, Chapters 8–12 present a series of case studies that describe real-life facilitation projects across a range of different subject areas and healthcare settings. These include projects in an acute hospital setting, in primary care, nursing homes and rural communities; what they have in common is that they all involved individuals working in facilitator roles to support and guide the implementation process. In our final Chapter 13, we compare across the five case studies to identify areas of similarity and difference and the key lessons learned about facilitation. This leads us into some final reflections about the i-PARIHS framework and our facilitation model, including setting out the issues that we think still need to be explored further.

Who should read this book and how should you use it?

By now you should have got an idea that this book is essentially a practical guide to facilitation and facilitator roles. Our aim is to make it relevant and useful to as wide an audience as possible across the range from novice to expert facilitators – those people with responsibility for introducing evidence and innovations into healthcare at a clinical, organisational and strategic level. We also believe that the ideas contained within the book will be useful to researchers working in the field of implementation science and knowledge translation in terms of designing studies and interventions that take account of the range of factors that could influence the processes and outcomes of implementation – and ensuring that the interventions introduced as part of a research study are sustainable once the research project has finished and the research team are no longer there.

We hope that those readers familiar with the PARIHS framework will find the book useful as a way to operationalise facilitation using a goal-focused approach and to reflect on our proposed revision to the original framework, paying greater attention to the recipients of the implementation process and the different levels of context within which implementation takes place. Given the complexities of implementation, it will never be possible to provide a blueprint of exactly 'how to do it'; however, we would like to think that this book maps out the key coordinates to think about and, most importantly, describes a practical range of strategies that can be used to facilitate implementation. As we said at the start of the chapter, facilitation is essentially a process of enabling others to act through structured and supported experiential learning. This is how we intend the book to be used – as a guide that can enable individuals and teams to become more knowledgeable, more confident and ultimately more proficient in implementing evidence-based innovation in practice.

References

Baskerville, N.B., Liddy, C. & Hogg, W. 2012. Systematic review and meta-analysis of practice facilitation within primary care settings. *Annals of Family Medicine*, 10, 63–74.
Chalmers, I. & Altman, D.G. 1995. *Systematic Reviews*. London: BMJ Publishing Group.
Cochrane, A.L. 1973. *Effectiveness and Efficiency: Random Reflections on Health Services*. London: Nuffield Provincial Hospitals Trust.

Cockburn, J., Ruth, D., Silagy, C., Dobbin, M., Reid, Y., Scollo, M. & Naccarella, L. 1992. Randomised trial of three approaches for marketing smoking cessation programmes to Australian general practitioners. *British Medical Journal*, 304, 691–4.

Davies, H., Nutley, S. & Walter, I. 2008. Why 'knowledge transfer' is misconceived for applied social research. *Journal of Health Services Research & Policy*, 13, 188–90.

Dawes, M., Davies, P., Gray, A., Mant, M., Seers, K. & Snowball, R. 1999. *Evidence-based Practice: A Primer for Health Care Professionals*. Edinburgh: Churchill Livingstone.

Deming, W.E. 2000. *Out of the Crisis*. Cambridge, MA: MIT Press.

DiCenso, A., Guyatt, G. & Ciliska, D. 2004. *Evidence-Based Nursing. A Guide to Clinical Practice*. St. Louis, MO: Elsevier Mosby.

Dopson, S. & Fitzgerald, L. 2005. *Knowledge to Action? Evidence-Based Health Care in Action*. New York: Oxford University Press.

Engels, Y., Van Den Hombergh, P., Mokkink, H., Van Den Hoogen, H., Van Den Bosch, W. & Grol, R. 2006. The effects of a team-based continuous quality improvement intervention on the management of primary care: a randomised controlled trial. *British Journal of General Practice*, 56, 781–7.

Evidence-based Medicine Working Group 1992. Evidence-based medicine. A new approach to teaching the practice of medicine. *Journal of the American Medical Association*, 268, 2420–5.

Ferlie, E., Fitzgerald, L. & Wood, M. 2000. Getting evidence into clinical practice: an organisational behaviour perspective. *Journal of Health Services Research & Policy*, 5, 96–102.

Fullard, E., Fowler, G. & Gray, M. 1984. Facilitating prevention in primary care. *British Medical Journal*, 289, 1585–7.

Greenhalgh, T., Robert, G., Macfarlane, F., Bate, P. & Kyriakidou, O. 2004. Diffussion of innovation in service organizations: systematic review and recommendations. *Milbank Quarterly*, 82, 581–629.

Grimshaw, J., Eccles, M., Lavis, J., Hill, S. & Squires, J. 2012. Knowledge translation of research findings. *Implementation Science*, 7, 50.

Grol, R. 2001. Successes and failures in the implementation of evidence-based guidelines for clinical practice. *Medical Care*, 39, 1146–54.

Heron, J. 1989. *The Facilitator's Handbook*. London: Kogan Page.

Hogan, C. 2002. *Understanding Facilitation: Theory and Principles*. London: Kogan Page.

Ingle, N. & Ingle, S. 1983. *Quality Circles in Service Industries — Comprehensive Guidelines for Increased Productivity and Efficiency*. New York: Prentice-Hall.

Institute for Healthcare Improvement 2003. The breakthrough series: IHI's collaborative model for achieving breakthrough improvement. IHI Innovation Series white paper. Boston: Institute for Healthcare Improvement.

Juran, J.M. & Godfrey, A.B. 1998. *Juran's Quality Handbook* (5th edn). New York: McGraw-Hill.

Liddy, C., Laferriere, D., Baskerville, B., Dahrouge, S., Knox, L. & Hogg, W. 2013. An overview of practice facilitation programs in Canada: current perspectives and future directions. *Healthcare Policy*, 8, 58–67.

Lomas, J. 2000. Using 'linkage and exchange' to move research into policy at a Canadian foundation. *Health Affairs*, 19, 236–40.

Mayo, E. 1933. *The Human Problems of an Industrial Civilization*. New York: Macmillan.

McCormack, B., Manley, K. & Titchen, A. 2013. *Practice Development in Nursing and Healthcare* (2nd edn). Chichester: John Wiley & Sons.

Morrell, C. & Harvey, G. 1999. *The Clinical Audit Handbook: Improving the Quality of Health Care*. London: Baillière Tindall.

Nutting, P.A., Crabtree, B.F., Stewart, E.E., Miller, W.L., Palmer, R.F., Stange, K.C. & Jaen, C.R. 2010. Effect of facilitation on practice outcomes in the National Demonstration Project model of the patient-centered medical home. *Annals of Family Medicine*, 8 Suppl 1, S33–44.

Palmer, A., Burns, S. & Bulman, C. 1994. *Reflective Practice in Nursing: The Growth of the Professional Practitioner*. Oxford: Blackwell.

Parchman, M., Noel, P., Culler, S., Lanham, H., Leykum, L., Romero, R. & Palmer, R. 2013. A randomized trial of practice facilitation to improve the delivery of chronic illness care in primary care: initial and sustained effects. *Implementation Science*, 8, 93.

Reason, P. & Rowan, J. 1981. *Human Inquiry: A Sourcebook of New Paradigm Research*. Chichester: John Wiley & Sons.

Rogers, C.R. 1969. *Freedom to Learn – A View of What Education Might Become*. Columbus, OH: Charles Merrill.

Rogers, E.M. 1995. *Diffusion of Innovations*. New York: The Free Press.

Royal College of Nursing 1990. *Quality Patient Care: The Dynamic Standard Setting System*. Harrow: Scutari.

Sackett, D.L., Rosenberg, W.M., Gray, J.A., Haynes, R.B. & Richardson, W.S. 1996. Evidence based medicine: What it is and what it isn't. *British Medical Journal*, 312, 71–2.

Van de Ven, A.H. & Johnson, P.E. 2006. Knowledge for theory and practice. *The Academy of Management Review*, 31, 802–21.

Walshe, K. & Rundall, T.G. 2001. Evidence-based management: From theory to practice in health care. *Milbank Quarterly*, 79, 429–57, iv–v.

2

FACILITATION AS THE ACTIVE INGREDIENT IN THE PARIHS FRAMEWORK

Gill Harvey and Alison Kitson

Introduction

This chapter presents a more detailed description of the Promoting Action on Research Implementation in Health Services framework – or PARIHS as it is commonly known – and in particular, the role of facilitation within the framework. We outline how and why the development of the PARIHS framework took place, including tracing back how our previous work on improving and developing practice shaped our thinking about implementation and facilitation. We then proceed to discuss the PARIHS framework in some detail, starting with the three elements that the framework proposed are fundamental to the successful implementation of evidence into practice, namely: the *evidence* to be implemented, the *context* in which implementation takes place and *facilitation* of the implementation process. Each of these elements is described, drawing on the work that we undertook to define the concepts of evidence, context and facilitation. This description is an important backdrop to the following chapter, in which we outline how the PARIHS framework has been applied over the last 15 years to guide and evaluate the implementation of evidence-based practice in healthcare. In turn, we will discuss how this has informed a proposed revision to PARIHS and influenced the development of the facilitation model that we are presenting in this book.

The development of the PARIHS framework

We have been working with the PARIHS framework since the late 1990s. The impetus for developing the framework came from collaboration with colleagues involved in trying to support the implementation of change and improvement in healthcare. Our collective experience suggested that the process was difficult, unpredictable, challenging and often messy, despite the models of research implementation and evidence-based decision-making in policy documents and the literature, which represented the process as a fairly straightforward linear series of steps that needed to be followed. Typically, these models suggested a rational process of moving from primary research through to evidence synthesis and dissemination; then to strategies to increase knowledge, awareness and skills in clinical staff (for example, through continuing education and professional development); and finally reinforcing the changes by way of ongoing audit and feedback. This 'push' model of implementing research into practice did not fit with our lived experience of implementation, where new ideas often arose from practice and where research evidence – however rigorous or robust it might be – could be challenged, contested and ignored by the people who were supposed to use it.

These experiences led us to question why the linear, rational models of research implementation seemed inadequate in terms of explaining what was really happening in practice and what would be a more realistic representation of the research implementation process. It is from these debates that the PARIHS framework developed. However, informing this discussion was 10–12 years' prior experience in developing, implementing and evaluating models of facilitation in our work on quality improvement, practice development and clinical leadership. Below we briefly summarise this early work to provide an overview of how and why our thinking about facilitation and implementing change has evolved over time, before moving on to the more detailed description of the PARIHS framework.

An evolving interest in facilitating change and improvement

To understand our views and beliefs about the facilitator's role in promoting evidence-based practice, it is first necessary to say a little bit about our own journey. Both nurses by background, we started working together in 1987 in a programme that was established within the professional organisation for nurses in the UK – the Royal College of Nursing (RCN) – to promote and maintain standards of nursing practice. Our early work was focused on developing and evaluating approaches to assure and improve nursing care quality. This included studying what approaches were being developed and used in other organisations and other countries (Harvey, 1991; Kitson and Harvey, 1991; Harvey and Kitson, 1996), as well as working on the development of our own model known as the Dynamic Standard Setting System, or DySSSy for short (Kendall and Kitson, 1986; Kitson, 1989; Royal College of Nursing, 1990). As the name implies, DySSSy started from a position that viewed the improvement of standards as an ongoing, iterative process – in contrast to the predominant models of nursing quality at the time, which tended to use pre-formulated measures and checklists. Key features of the DySSSy method were its emphasis on practitioners defining, evaluating and improving their own standards of care in a 'bottom-up' and incremental way. This was achieved through applying a problem-focused and systems-based, structure–process–outcome approach (Donabedian, 2005) to analyse the inputs and processes needed to achieve particular outcomes. To support local practitioners working within improvement teams, the DySSSy method advocated a network of facilitators: local facilitators to help with the implementation of standards and audit in practice; key facilitators to oversee and coordinate the quality programme, including the provision of education and training for local facilitators; expert facilitators to introduce and plan strategic level quality improvement. Box 2.1 provides the definitions of facilitation used with the DySSSy system and summarises the roles at the different levels of facilitation.

BOX 2.1   FACILITATION AND FACILITATOR ROLES WITHIN THE DYNAMIC STANDARD SETTING SYSTEM (DySSSy)

- *Facilitation*: The process by which a group is helped to achieve its purpose by a facilitator who promotes the improvement of team dynamics and the active involvement of all group members.
- *Facilitator*: An individual who works with groups to help them develop team dynamics by improving group processes and achieving active involvement of all group members in the content of the team's efforts.
- *Expert facilitator*: Equivalent to an external change agent whose job is to introduce the quality programme into the organisation, develop training courses, act as an external consultant, update on methodology and help set the organisational structure for quality.
- *Key facilitator*: The insider or internal change agent with a central role in coordinating organisation-wide quality activities, responsible for initiating the quality programme at a local level, training staff and generally keeping everything going.
- *Local facilitator*: Identified by the key facilitator to support quality improvement activity at the local level on an ongoing basis. The local facilitator also helps the key facilitator to spread the initiative throughout the organisation.

As the DySSSy method gained in popularity and use, we established facilitator development programmes and networks. We also gained increasing knowledge about the facilitator role and function in quality improvement and audit through an ongoing programme of research and development (Harvey, 1991; Kitson et al., 1994; Harvey and Kitson, 1996; Morrell et al., 1997). These studies highlighted the central role of the facilitator in enabling and supporting improvement, for example, in relation to establishing the willingness and motivation of clinical staff to get involved in quality improvement. This was greater when the staff respected the person in the facilitator role and viewed them as credible. Key qualities that appeared to be important in a successful facilitator included good communication skills, an ability to empower others, a willingness to change the status quo, enthusiasm and a commitment to improving patient care (Morrell et al., 1997).

This growing interest in developing the knowledge base of facilitation was also informed by other programmes of work within the RCN, including those on practice development and clinical leadership. For example, in parallel to the work on standards and quality, initiatives were underway to develop, refine and evaluate models and frameworks for practice development. These began from the perspective of promoting more person-centred care through enabling the development and empowerment of practitioners, accompanied by cultural change within the care setting to sustain the growth in practice, as the following definition illustrates.

> Practice development is a continuous process of improvement towards increased effectiveness in person-centred care, through the enabling of nurses and health care teams to transform the culture and context of care. It is enabled and supported by facilitators committed to a systematic, rigorous and continuous process of emancipatory change.
>
> *(McCormack et al., 1999, p.256)*

Within this process, skilled facilitation, located within a philosophy of emancipatory change was seen to be essential. As such, this approach to practice development firmly located itself within a critical social science perspective and the facilitator's role was that of a 'critical companion' (Titchen and McGinley, 2003), using a range of critical dialogue and reflective practice skills to support practitioners on an experiential learning journey. Since these early developments, work on practice development and the facilitator role within the development process has grown significantly, with the establishment of an International Practice Development Collaborative (IPDC), an international practice development journal and regular facilitation summer schools (see http://www.fons.org/library/about-ipdc.aspx for further information).

As the description of practice development illustrates, the approach to facilitation is rather different in focus than that we described in the work on standards and quality. Different interpretations of the facilitator role and differences in facilitation methods are a feature throughout the literature – and this is something that we will explore in more detail as we move through the book. To illustrate this, it is useful to briefly consider a third area of work that developed within the RCN, again employing facilitation methods to support the development of clinical leaders. The Clinical Leadership Programme commenced in 1994, in response to a recognised need to develop the leadership role of ward/unit leaders in providing quality patient care (Cunningham and Kitson, 2000a, 2000b). Through a collaborative action research project with ward leaders, a framework to underpin clinical leadership development was produced. This framework comprised five themes, representing the areas where nurses needed to develop in order to become patient-centred clinical leaders, namely: learning to manage self; creating effective relationships within teams; maintaining a consistent patient focus; networking; and developing political awareness. A range of interventions were used to support learning and development across these five themes, including personal development and mentorship, action learning, patient stories and observation of care, team building and service improvement projects. Central to the delivery and support of the programme was a network of facilitators, working in an external–internal facilitator relationship, with designated roles of lead facilitator, regional facilitator and local facilitator (Large et al., 2005). Within this model, facilitation was defined as follows:

> Facilitation means to make things simpler. . . . this means working with groups of individuals to enable them to achieve their potential and become skilled at how to learn again. Facilitation is seen as an integral part of leadership development. On the [clinical leadership] programme, each of the local facilitators has a considerable amount of experiential learning opportunities to develop their role as facilitators, and in turn become very strong role models to the clinical leaders participating in the programme.
>
> *(Large et al., 2005, p.6)*

As indicated in the definition, the emphasis was on a cascade model of facilitation with the lead and regional facilitators providing an external source of expertise and support via a structured development programme for local facilitators, who in turn were facilitating development and learning among their own clinical teams. Overall, the approach of the Clinical Leadership Programme combined elements of both the quality improvement and practice development initiatives, with a clear focus on improving specific aspects of patient care while at the same time supporting the personal development of leaders through experiential and reflective learning.

These examples describe work on facilitation that commenced within the same organisation, although the individuals involved subsequently moved into new posts in different organisations, where they continued to develop their respective areas of interest. However, in the earlier stages, the programmes of work on quality improvement, practice development and clinical leadership were being undertaken in parallel, each with their own interpretation and application of the facilitation process and facilitator role. This enabled a considerable amount of discussion and shared learning across the different project teams – not necessarily to reach a shared view, but to explore areas of similarity and difference and at times agree to disagree! Perhaps more than anything what this learning across different projects and different approaches demonstrated was that there is not one right approach to facilitation. Depending on the focus and purpose of the project or activity that is being facilitated, it is quite likely that a different set of facilitation methods and styles will be needed – a characteristic that we aimed to reflect in the PARIHS framework and that we will discuss in more detail in subsequent chapters of the book.

At this point, it is also important to highlight that we were exploring issues related to developing and improving practice at a time when interest and activity around the field of evidence-based practice in healthcare began to emerge. Building on the work we had undertaken in standards and audit, we became involved in developing national clinical guidelines in topic areas such as venous leg ulcers, pressure ulcers and pain in children, while at the same time paying attention to how the guidelines could be implemented in practice. So, for example, we developed implementation resources to accompany the clinical guidelines and established national audit programmes – again built around a model of facilitation – to support the processes of implementation and evaluation in practice (Morrell et al., 2001). It was the developing policy and practice focus on evidence-based healthcare, combined with a deep-rooted interest in issues of implementation and how to facilitate practice change and improvement, that provided the springboard for the development of the PARIHS framework.

The PARIHS framework

The starting premise of PARIHS is that the successful implementation of research evidence is a function of the interplay of the evidence to be implemented (its nature and how it fits with clinical, patient and local experience), the context in which implementation is to take place (in terms of the culture and general receptiveness to new ideas) and the way in which the process is facilitated (by whom and in what way). In turn, each of these elements of evidence, context and facilitation is seen to comprise several sub-elements, resulting in a picture of implementation that is multi-dimensional and dynamic.

We will explain in some more detail what the elements look like and how we think they fit together. But first, a continuation of the story about how the framework came into being. As noted above, we were working within a diverse team of researchers, practice developers and improvement facilitators, all grappling with similar issues around the complexities of implementation and how best to achieve it in practice. Through discussing and sharing our experiences, the first version of the PARIHS framework was inductively developed and published in 1998 (Kitson et al., 1998). This produced a working hypothesis that suggested the most successful implementation of research evidence into practice was likely to occur when the research evidence was high (defined as rigorous and robust research that aligned with clinical experience and patient preferences), the context for implementation was high (defined as a receptive culture with supportive leadership and routine monitoring of quality and performance) and facilitation was high (defined as a facilitator in an appropriate role with the right set of characteristics and a flexible style of working). Different combinations of the evidence, context and facilitation triad were tested using retrospective case study data from a number of implementation and evaluation studies to provide initial empirical support for the framework. Comparing the findings across these studies – which are described in more detail in the original PARIHS publication (Kitson et al., 1998) – also suggested that facilitation appeared to be a key variable within the implementation process.

From this point, we continued to undertake more development, evaluation and refinement of the PARIHS framework. This included undertaking detailed concept analyses of the core elements of evidence, context and facilitation within the framework, alongside a case study evaluation of two implementation projects to compare real-life experiences of implementation against the PARIHS dimensions. The result was some modifications to the original PARIHS framework (Rycroft-Malone et al., 2002), plus the identification of questions and issues that have informed our ongoing interest and study of implementation and facilitation in relation to evidence-based healthcare. Box 2.2 provides a summary of the key references documenting the development and testing of the PARIHS framework. We will now describe the characteristics of evidence, context and facilitation as defined in the 2002 version of PARIHS.

BOX 2.2   REFERENCES TRACING THE DEVELOPMENT AND TESTING OF THE PARIHS FRAMEWORK (1996–2004)

Kitson, A., Harvey, G. & McCormack, B. 1998. Enabling the implementation of evidence based practice: a conceptual framework. *Quality in Health Care*, 7(3), 149–58.

Rycroft-Malone, J., Kitson, A., Harvey, G., McCormack, B., Seers, K., Titchen, A. & Estabrookes, C. 2002. Ingredients for change: revisiting a conceptual framework. *Quality and Safety in Healthcare*, 11(2), 174–80.

Harvey, G., Loftus-Hills, A., Rycroft-Malone, J., Titchen, A., Kitson, A., McCormack, B. & Seers, K. 2002. Getting evidence into practice: the role and function of facilitation. *Journal of Advanced Nursing*, 37(6), 577–88.

McCormack, B., Kitson, A., Harvey, G., Rycroft-Malone, J., Titchen, A. & Seers, K. 2002. Getting evidence into practice: the meaning of context. *Journal of Advanced Nursing*, 38(1), 94–104.

Rycroft-Malone, J., Seers, K., Titchen, A., Harvey, G., Kitson, A. & McCormack, B. 2004. What counts as evidence in evidence-based practice? *Journal of Advanced Nursing*, 47(1), 81–90.

Rycroft-Malone, J., Harvey, G., Seers, K., Kitson, A., McCormack, B. & Titchen, A. 2004. An exploration of the factors that influence the implementation of evidence into practice. *Journal of Clinical Nursing*, 13, 913–924.

Kitson, A., Rycroft-Malone, J., Harvey, G., McCormack, B., Seers, K. & Titchen, A. 2008. Evaluating the successful implementation of evidence into practice using the PARIHS framework: theoretical and practical challenges. *Implementation Science*, 3, 1.

Evidence

The *evidence* element within PARIHS was examined through a process of concept analysis (Rycroft-Malone et al., 2004b) and an empirical study of implementing evidence into clinical practice (Rycroft-Malone et al., 2004a). The results suggested that evidence comprised a number of sub-elements, namely: research, clinical experience, patient experience and local

TABLE 2.1 Attributes of 'high' (strong) evidence

Dimension of evidence	Attributes at the 'high', end of the continuum
Research	• Well-conceived, designed and executed research • Seen as one part of a decision • Valued as evidence • Lack of certainty acknowledged • Social construction acknowledged • Judged as relevant • Importance weighted • Conclusions drawn
Clinical experience	• Clinical experience and expertise reflected upon and tested by individuals and groups • Consensus within similar groups • Valued as evidence • Seen as one part of the decision • Judged as relevant • Importance weighted • Conclusions drawn
Patient experience	• Valued as evidence • Multiple biographies used • Partnerships with healthcare professionals • Seen as one part of a decision • Judged as relevant • Importance weighted • Conclusions drawn
Local experience	• Valued as evidence • Collected and analysed systematically and rigorously • Evaluated and reflected upon • Conclusions drawn

Source: After Rycroft-Malone et al. (2004a, 2004b).

information. Thus, although the PARIHS framework was principally concerned with the implementation of research evidence, a key message was that research alone did not determine whether it is implemented in practice. Rather, research was seen to sit alongside clinical, patient and local experience and decisions about implementing research were dependent on these other sources of evidence. Adding another layer of detail, the PARIHS framework then suggested that each of the four sub-elements of evidence could be represented on a continuum from low to high. At the 'high' end of the continuum research was viewed as rigorous and robust, consensus of clinical opinion had been achieved and accepted as a valid source of evidence, patients had been actively involved and their views valued and local information had been systematically analysed and evaluated. The PARIHS framework proposed that the more these four sub-elements of evidence aligned towards the high end of the continuum, the stronger the evidence to underpin implementation (Table 2.1).

This view of evidence as complex and multi-faceted aligns with much of the wider literature on evidence and evidence-based practice. Increasingly, it is recognised that the more traditional views of evidence as something that is derived from research and, as such, is concrete and irrefutable do not represent the reality of healthcare and clinical practice. Historically, the more objective definitions of evidence stem from the biomedical sciences, where research evidence is produced as a result of highly controlled experiments. The formal, explicit knowledge produced as a result tends to be privileged over more practical and tacit 'know-how' knowledge (Harvey, 2013). A contrasting view is put forward from a social science perspective; here knowledge is seen to be socially situated, encompassing both explicit and tacit dimensions and – crucially – subject to influence by the social and contextual environment (Greenhalgh and Wieringa, 2011). Empirical studies tracking the implementation journey of evidence-based innovations in practice tend to confirm this broader, social science view of evidence, demonstrating that however robust the research evidence is perceived to be, it is typically subject to processes of local sense-making, contestation and adaptation (Dopson and Fitzgerald, 2005). This multi-faceted and negotiated nature of evidence is something that the PARIHS definition and dimensions of evidence attempted to reflect.

Context

The second element of the PARIHS framework is *context*, defined as the 'environment or setting in which the proposed change is to be implemented' (Kitson et al., 1998, p.150). The context dimension was also analysed in depth as part of the development of the PARIHS framework (McCormack et al., 2002) and the key sub-elements identified: culture, leadership and (continuous) evaluation and learning. As with the evidence dimension, these sub-elements were represented on a continuum from high to low and characteristics of a 'high' or supportive context for implementation were identified (Table 2.2). At a general level, a receptive context for implementation was seen to be one where there was transparency of decision-making, appropriate human, financial and support resources, where the planned change fitted with strategic priorities and where prevailing power and authority relationships were supportive of innovation. More specifically, a culture supportive of implementation was defined as one with clearly defined beliefs and values, which valued individuals within the organisation (staff and clients), had clearly defined roles and responsibilities, promoted teamwork and collaboration, and recognised and rewarded achievement. A transformational style of leadership was seen to be important to creating a supportive context; in other words, leadership that was democratic, inclusive, enabling and empowering. Finally, PARIHS proposed that an organisational orientation to evaluation and learning was a vital component of the context. Thus, organisations that systematically paid attention to performance at the individual, team and system level and which used multiple and varied sources of data (both quantitative and qualitative) to make judgements about performance, were seen to create a more supportive context for implementation. As with the evidence dimension, the underlying assumption was that the more the sub-elements of culture, leadership and evaluation aligned towards the high end of the continuum, the more supportive the context for implementation would be.

Recognition of the importance of context in determining the processes and outcomes of implementation has received increasing recognition in the literature over recent years. Accounts of projects that have attempted to implement evidence, for example, in the form of clinical guidelines or through improvement initiatives, typically conclude that 'context matters' (Kaplan et al., 2010; Bate et al., 2014). Contextual factors at both the immediate project level

TABLE 2.2 Attributes of a 'high' (supportive) context

Dimension of context	Attributes at the 'high', end of the continuum
Resources and infrastructure	• Physical, social, professional, cultural, structural and system boundaries clearly defined and acknowledged • Appropriate and transparent decision-making processes • Resources – human, financial, equipment – allocated • Initiative fits with strategic goals and is a key practice/patient issue

Culture	• Able to define culture(s) in terms of prevailing values/beliefs
	• Values individual staff and clients
	• Promotes a learning organisation philosophy
	• Consistency between individual's role and experience in terms of valuing:
	   o relationships with others
	   o teamwork
	   o power and authority
	   o rewards/recognition

Leadership	• Transformational leadership • Role clarity • Effective teamwork • Effective organisational structures • Democratic inclusive decision-making processes • Enabling/empowering approach to teaching/learning/managing
Evaluation	• Feedback on individual, team and system performance • Use of multiple sources of information on performance • Use of multiple methods to evaluate clinical processes and outcomes, economic outcomes, user experiences, etc. • Routine use of data feedback and monitoring

Source: Adapted from McCormack et al. (2002), Rycroft-Malone et al.(2004a).

and the wider organisational or health system level can influence the way that implementation projects play out in practice. Various instruments have been developed to assess contextual factors and the potential barriers to implementation, with a corresponding emphasis on the need to tailor implementation strategies to the local context (Wensing et al., 2010).

However, there is generally less guidance on what to do at a practical level to deal with the influence exerted by context and achieve the right sort of tailoring within individual implementation projects. This is where the PARIHS framework suggested facilitation as a vital ingredient in implementation – providing an active and interactive process to assess and respond to contextual factors when planning and managing the implementation process.

Facilitation

As discussed earlier in the chapter, when we developed the PARIHS framework, we drew initially on our own experiences of facilitating change through quality improvement and practice development initiatives. This influenced how we incorporated facilitation into PARIHS in a number of ways.

First, we positioned facilitation as the active component of the PARIHS framework with an individual in a designated role as facilitator applying a range of (facilitation) methods and processes to enable the process of implementing evidence into practice. Evidence, in this sense, could be an established 'product', such as a clinical guideline, or it could be a problem identified in the practice setting that required an evidence-based approach to finding solutions and implementing improvement. In either case, the facilitator's role was to work with relevant stakeholders to identify and/or examine the available evidence and find strategies to support the implementation of that evidence within the specific local context. So in the case of an existing guideline, the focus might be on establishing the extent to which the evidence presented in the guideline matched local, clinical and patient experience and agreeing a consensus on what to implement and how. By contrast, when the starting point was a clinical problem or topic for improvement, the initial emphasis was likely to be on searching for available sources of evidence and then collating and synthesising these in a way that was appropriate and applicable to the local problem and context. In both cases, the facilitator had to navigate and negotiate between the evidence and the local context in an iterative and interactive way.

Second, we proposed that the facilitation concept encompasses a broad range of roles and activities that range from explicitly supporting the achievement of a specific goal to a more general focus on transforming individuals, teams, organisations and health systems to create a culture that is more open and receptive to change and improvement. In our concept analysis of facilitation (Harvey et al., 2002), we positioned these differing roles and interpretations of facilitation along a continuum from task-focused to holistic facilitation (Figure 2.1). At the left-hand side of the continuum the facilitation process was predominantly focused on achieving the goals of the task (for example, the implementation of a particular clinical guideline), something that could be achieved through providing practical and technical help with the implementation process. This type of facilitation is often provided by external facilitators who have periodic contact with the individuals and team responsible for implementation. As a result, the facilitation approach is relatively low in intensity and can target a number of different teams or organisations at the same time.

In contrast, the right-hand side of the continuum was described as a more holistic approach to facilitation. Here the focus was not specifically on the task, but on releasing the potential of individuals so that they could achieve the task. This involved a wider focus on issues relating to culture, power and politics within organisations and teams. The typical model of facilitation is external facilitators working in partnership with internal facilitators, providing them with opportunities for critical reflection and development; ultimately, the aim is to empower internal facilitators to achieve change, including addressing the contextual issues that might impact

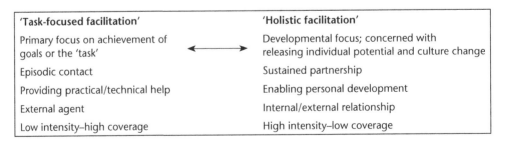

'Task-focused facilitation'	'Holistic facilitation'
Primary focus on achievement of goals or the 'task'	Developmental focus; concerned with releasing individual potential and culture change
Episodic contact	Sustained partnership
Providing practical/technical help	Enabling personal development
External agent	Internal/external relationship
Low intensity–high coverage	High intensity–low coverage

FIGURE 2.1 A continuum of facilitation. After Harvey et al. (2002)

upon implementation. This requires a more resource-intensive facilitation strategy involving a sustained partnership between the internal and external facilitator.

Third, depending on the focus of the facilitation activity, we suggested that the facilitator's role and the corresponding skills required to perform the role would also differ along a continuum, with the more task/goal-focused approach requiring technical and project management type skills and the holistic/enabling approach requiring skills such as critical reflection and co-counselling (Figure 2.2).

Finally, we recognised that in practice, facilitation activities would rarely be located at a fixed point on the continuum and that 'hybrid' facilitator roles could exist, with facilitators undertaking both task and enabling activities at different points in time within the same project. This would typically be the case where facilitators were focused on supporting the achievement of particular goals or objectives, yet at the same time needed to pay attention to the process by which those goals were agreed, actioned and achieved.

Essentially the PARIHS framework suggested that the facilitator role and the facilitation process provided a way of tailoring implementation strategies according to the evidence to be implemented and factors within the local context that might hinder or support implementation. Figure 2.3 illustrates this in relation to different ways that evidence and context might present according to where each concept sits on a high to low continuum (Kitson et al., 2008). For example, quadrant F1 on the diagram represents a situation where the evidence is seen to be 'high'. This could be a situation where a national clinical guideline exists that has been developed with appropriate professional and patient involvement. The guideline addresses an issue that has been identified as a priority by the health system at a local level and there is broad professional consensus that it represents good practice. However, the context is weak and not receptive to change as judged by the dimensions of culture, leadership and evaluation. Past attempts at introducing change and innovation have been mostly unsuccessful for a number of reasons. Relationships between clinicians (notably the doctors) and managers are difficult and often confrontational, largely because of the target-driven way in which the organisation has been run in the past. This has led to many staff feeling that change is imposed, with a lack of guidance or support around what needs to be done and no apparent time or resources to do the work required. In this situation, the facilitator's role will be particularly concerned with addressing these contextual issues – exploring the reasons for resistance in some more depth, identifying strategies and resources to manage the implementation process, securing senior management support to the agreed plan of implementation and establishing clinical buy-in to the project through creating effective processes for staff involvement, participation and communication.

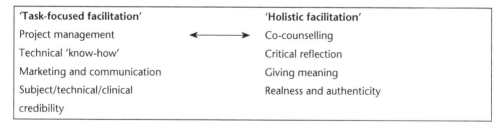

FIGURE 2.2 Facilitator roles and skills along the continuum. After Harvey et al. (2002)

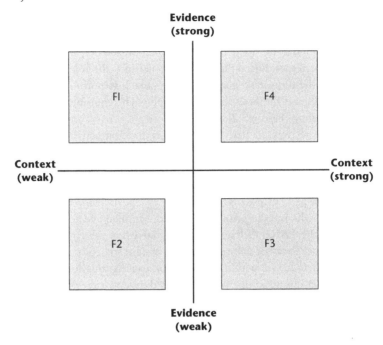

FI = facilitation approach to be adopted in situation of strong evidence, weak context

F2 = facilitation approach to be adopted in situation of weak evidence, weak context

F3 = facilitation approach to be adopted in situation of weak evidence, strong context

F4 = facilitation approach to be adopted in situation of strong evidence, strong context

FIGURE 2.3 Facilitation approaches in relation to evidence and context. After Kitson et al. (2008)

By contrast, in a situation where the context was generally supportive of change, but the evidence weak or viewed differently by different stakeholder groups (situation F3), the facilitator's role would be more concerned with building consensus around the evidence to be implemented, for example, by bringing together the different stakeholder groups (such as clinicians, patients, managers and commissioners) to review the evidence, share their own experiences and reach agreement on the changes to be made. Different scenarios could also be envisaged for quadrants F2 (weak evidence, weak context) and F4 (strong evidence, strong context). The key point is that facilitation represented the element of the PARIHS framework that could flex and adapt to meet the specific circumstances of implementation. Adopting this view of facilitation raised a number of questions in relation to developing and applying the facilitator role in practice. For example, is the implication that facilitators need to be able to occupy any point on the facilitation continuum depending on the specific needs of the project and the organisational setting in which they are working? And, if so, what does this mean in terms of identifying and preparing individuals to take on the facilitator role? Is it realistic, for example, to expect a novice facilitator to possess – or be able to develop – the full skill-set needed to move up and down the continuum before they take on the facilitator role in practice? And where and how do facilitators begin when they start working with a group attempting to implement evidence-based practice for the first time?

These are all questions that we have deliberated, discussed and reflected upon as we have applied our thinking about facilitation and the PARIHS framework in various implementation projects over the last 10–15 years – and the answers to which have helped to inform our description of the facilitator's role in this book. In presenting answers to these questions, our approach is essentially a pragmatic one. The conclusion that we have come to, both from our own experiences and from reviewing relevant empirical and theoretical literature on implementation science, is that facilitation is a skilled and complex process. However, it is a process – and a role – that has to be operationalised in the real-life environment of healthcare where resources are finite, time is pressured and change and re-organisation are ever-present. In Chapter 4, we will outline a facilitation model that we think is pragmatic and practical, but which recognises the complexities of implementation. Before we describe this model, we will first re-visit the PARIHS framework to describe why and how we think it should be revised.

Summary

This chapter has traced the evolution and development of the PARIHS framework as a way of conceptualising the factors that influence the successful implementation of evidence-based practice in healthcare. In the next chapter we will look at how PARIHS has been applied over the last 15 years within the field of implementation and implementation research. This has raised questions about the construction of the framework itself and about how to move from a conceptual framework to a more operational model. We will consider the published critiques of PARIHS and draw on a range of experiential, empirical and theoretical literature to explain why we think it is a good time to re-visit the original PARIHS framework. Having set out a rationale for a revised framework, described as the integrated-PARIHS (i-PARIHS) framework, we will then apply this in subsequent chapters to present an operational model of facilitation.

It is as a result of the ongoing learning about PARIHS and about implementing evidence-based practice more generally – both from our own and others' experiences – that the facilitation model we are presenting in this book has developed and taken shape. In particular, our concern has been to produce a model that demonstrates in a very practical way how facilitation can function as an active intervention to respond to the requirements of different implementation projects and tailor interventions appropriately to the particular project, the people involved and the setting in which they work.

References

Bate, P., Robert, G., Fulop, N., Ovretveit, J. & Dixon-Woods, M. 2014. *Perspectives on Context. A Selection of Essays Considering the Role of Context in Successful Quality Improvement.* London: Health Foundation.

Cunningham, G. & Kitson, A. 2000a. An evaluation of the RCN Clinical Leadership Development Programme: part 1. *Nursing Standard*, 15, 34–7.

Cunningham, G. & Kitson, A. 2000b. An evaluation of the RCN Clinical Leadership Development Programme: part 2. *Nursing Standard*, 15, 34–40.

Donabedian, A. 2005. Evaluating the quality of medical care. 1966. *Milbank Quarterly*, 83, 691–729.

Dopson, S. & Fitzgerald, L. 2005. *Knowledge to Action? Evidence-Based Health Care in Action*. New York: Oxford University Press.

Greenhalgh, T. & Wieringa, S. 2011. Is it time to drop the 'knowledge translation' metaphor? A critical literature review. *Journal of the Royal Society of Medicine*, 104, 501–509.

Harvey, G. 1991. An evaluation of approaches to assessing the quality of nursing care using (predetermined) quality assurance tools. *Journal of Advanced Nursing*, 16, 277–86.

Harvey, G. 2013. The many meanings of evidence: implications for the translational science agenda in healthcare. *International Journal of Health Policy and Management*, 1, 187–8.

Harvey, G. & Kitson, A. 1996. Achieving improvement through quality: an evaluation of key factors in the implementation process. *Journal of Advanced Nursing*, 24, 185–95.

Harvey, G., Loftus-Hills, A., Rycroft-Malone, J., Titchen, A., Kitson, A., McCormack, B. & Seers, K. 2002. Getting evidence into practice: the role and function of facilitation. *Journal of Advanced Nursing*, 37, 577–88.

Kaplan, H.C., Brady, P.W., Dritz, M.C., Hooper, D.K., Linam, W.M., Froehle, C.M. & Margolis, P. 2010. The influence of context on quality improvement success in health care: a systematic review of the literature. *Milbank Quarterly*, 88, 500–59.

Kendall, H. & Kitson, A. 1986. Quality assurance – rest assured. *Nursing Times*, 82, 29–31.

Kitson, A. 1989. *A Framework for Quality: A Patient-Centred Approach to Quality Assurance in Health Care*. Harrow, Middlesex: Scutari.

Kitson, A. & Harvey, G. 1991. *Bibliography of Nursing Quality Assurance and Standards of Care 1932–1987*. Harrow, Middlesex: Scutari.

Kitson, A., Harvey, G., Hyndman, S. & Sindhu, F. 1994. *The Impact of a Nursing Quality Assurance Approach, the Dynamic Standard Setting System (DySSSy) on Nursing Practice and Patient Outcomes (The ODySSSy Project)*. Oxford: National Institute for Nursing.

Kitson, A., Harvey, G. & McCormack, B. 1998. Enabling the implementation of evidence based practice: a conceptual framework. *Quality in Health Care*, 7, 149–59.

Kitson, A., Rycroft-Malone, J., Harvey, G., McCormack, B., Seers, K. & Titchen, A. 2008. Evaluating the successful implementation of evidence into practice using the PARIHS framework: theoretical and practical challenges (2008). *Implementation Science*, 3, 1.

Large, S., Macleod, A., Cunningham, G. & Kitson, A. 2005. *A Multiple-Case Study Evaluation of the RCN Clinical Leadership Programme in England*. London: Royal College of Nursing.

McCormack, B., Manley, K., Kitson, A., Titchen, A. & Harvey, G. 1999. Towards practice development: a vision in reality or a reality without vision? *Journal of Nursing Management*, 7, 255–64.

McCormack, B., Kitson, A., Harvey, G., Rycroft-Malone, J., Titchen, A. & Seers, K. 2002. Getting evidence into practice: the meaning of 'context'. *Journal of Advanced Nursing*, 38, 94–104.

Morrell, C., Harvey, G. & Kitson, A. 1997. Practitioner based quality improvement: a review of the Royal College of Nursing's Dynamic Standard Setting System. *Quality in Health Care*, 6, 29–34.

Morrell, C., Liao, X.H., Cheater, F., Dealey, C. & Nelson, A. 2001. The management of venous leg ulcers: a project to improve care. *Nursing Standard*, 15, 68–73.

Royal College of Nursing 1990. *Quality Patient Care: The Dynamic Standard Setting System*. Harrow, Middlesex: Scutari.

Rycroft-Malone, J., Kitson, A., Harvey, G., McCormack, B., Seers, K., Titchen, A. & Estabrooks, C. 2002. Ingredients for change: revisiting a conceptual framework. *Quality and Safety in Health Care*, 11, 174–80.

Rycroft-Malone, J., Harvey, G., Seers, K., Kitson, A., McCormack, B. & Titchen, A. 2004a. An exploration of the factors that influence the implementation of evidence into practice. *Journal of Clinical Nursing*, 13, 913–24.

Rycroft-Malone, J., Seers, K., Titchen, A., Harvey, G., Kitson, A. & McCormack, B. 2004b. What counts as evidence in evidence-based practice? *Journal of Advanced Nursing*, 47, 81–90.

Titchen, A. & McGinley, M. 2003. Facilitating practitioner research through critical companionship. *Nursing Times Research*, 8, 115–31.

Wensing, M., Bosch, M. & Grol, R. 2010. Developing and selecting interventions for translating knowledge to action. *Canadian Medical Association Journal*, 182, E85–E88.

3

PARIHS RE-VISITED

Introducing the i-PARIHS framework

Gill Harvey and Alison Kitson

Introduction

In this chapter we review how the PARIHS framework has been applied over the last 15 years to guide and evaluate the implementation of evidence-based practice in healthcare. We also consider how PARIHS compares to other implementation frameworks and models by drawing on some recently completed reviews within the implementation science literature. We then summarise the key theories that have been influential in informing and developing our understanding and practice of facilitation since the original development of the PARIHS framework. Building on this preceding discussion, we will explain why and how we have revised the PARIHS framework from its original conception to what we are now calling the integrated-PARIHS or i-PARIHS framework. This revised framework includes a re-conceptualisation of the constructs to be considered during implementation and is more explicitly underpinned by relevant theories of innovation, behavioural and organisational change and improvement. By bringing together our own and others' experiential and empirical evidence of using PARIHS with the wider theoretical literature, our intention has been to produce a more integrated conceptual framework to guide implementation. The core elements of i-PARIHS will be described, namely: the innovation to be implemented; the intended recipients of the innovation; the internal and external context in which implementation takes place; and the facilitation approach that is required to operationalise the framework.

Application of the PARIHS framework in implementation and implementation research

Since its original publication, the PARIHS framework has been applied widely across a range of different topics within different organisational settings and at different organisational levels, as the case study chapters later in the book will illustrate. A 2010 critical synthesis of the literature on PARIHS reviewed 24 published papers and noted that it was most commonly used as a heuristic, for example, in terms of providing an organising framework for analysing and reporting study findings or for framing the development of survey instruments (Helfrich et al., 2010). This was seen to reflect the intuitive appeal and relevance of the framework among users working in the field of implementation, notably because it recognised the complexity of implementation and the influence of context. This suggested a level of face and content validity for the framework. However, the review also highlighted perceived limitations of PARIHS, including the relatively limited evaluation of the framework in prospective implementation studies, the lack of clarity about the relationships between the elements and sub-elements of PARIHS, a predominant focus on the facilitator role, with less attention on the facilitation process, and the lack of a clear definition of successful implementation. Building on this synthesis, a revised PARIHS framework was proposed (Stetler et al., 2011), with more detailed guidance on how to interpret and apply the key elements of evidence, context and facilitation in practice.

Since the review by Helfrich and colleagues, further papers describing the application of the PARIHS framework have been published. A repeat search using the same databases and search terms as those applied in the 2010 review suggests a further 40 plus papers on PARIHS have been published in the last 5 years. This indicates the continuing interest in the framework, although studies that apply the framework prospectively remain limited. One exception to this is a recently reported trial that used PARIHS to design a study on the implementation of evidence-based guidelines for peri-operative fasting (Rycroft-Malone et al., 2012). From their analysis, the authors suggested that the framework failed to acknowledge the prominent role that individuals could play in determining the processes and outcomes of implementation by way of their interaction with evidence and context. This led the study authors to suggest that individuals should be a discrete element for consideration within future iterations of the PARIHS framework (Rycroft-Malone et al., 2013). A similar finding is apparent in some of the reviews that have compared PARIHS to other implementation frameworks and models, as we will discuss in the following section.

PARIHS compared to other implementation frameworks and models

PARIHS is one of a range of frameworks and models that have been developed to inform and guide the implementation of evidence-based practice. We do not intend to describe the other frameworks and models in detail – not least because there are so many alternative ones to consider. For example, a recent review in the *American Journal of Preventive Medicine* looked at commonly cited dissemination and implementation models that had been published up until the year 2011 and identified 61 different models (Tabak et al., 2012). For a description and summary of some of the main frameworks and models that have been used in healthcare, we would recommend readers to a book written specifically on this subject and edited by Jo Rycroft-Malone and Tracey Bucknall: *Models and Frameworks for Implementing Evidence-Based Practice: Linking Evidence to Action* (Rycroft-Malone and Bucknall, 2010).

For the purposes of this chapter, we are really interested in how PARIHS compares to the other frameworks and models that are available and what insights this provides in terms of the perceived strengths and weaknesses of PARIHS. We will do this by considering some recently published reviews on implementation theories, frameworks and models.

Damschroder and colleagues developed the Consolidated Framework for Implementation Research (CFIR) (Damschroder et al., 2009) as an overarching typology of the key constructs that influence implementation across multiple contexts. The CFIR was developed by reviewing published theories, frameworks and models of implementation, building on an earlier review that had been conducted on the diffusion, dissemination and implementation of innovations in health service delivery and organisation (Greenhalgh et al., 2004). Nineteen theories, frameworks and models were considered in the development of the CFIR, one of which was PARIHS. Comparison across the different theories, frameworks and models identified five major domains or categories of factors that influenced implementation and were described as: intervention characteristics; outer setting; inner setting; characteristics of the individuals involved; and the process of implementation (Table 3.1).

An alternative approach was adopted in the development of the Theoretical Domains Framework (TDF), which aims to assess the factors that influence healthcare professionals' behaviour and can be used to examine and understand potential barriers to implementation. The TDF was developed as an integrative framework of theories of behaviour change (Michie et al., 2005). This was in response to the growing interest in using existing theories to inform the implementation of evidence-based healthcare, alongside the recognition of the vast number

TABLE 3.1 The Consolidated Framework for Implementation Research

Domain	*Constructs related to the domain*
Intervention characteristics	<ul><li>Intervention source</li><li>Evidence strength and quality</li><li>Relative advantage</li><li>Adaptability</li><li>Trialability</li><li>Complexity</li><li>Design quality and packaging</li><li>Cost</li></ul>
Outer setting	<ul><li>Patient needs and resources</li><li>Cosmopolitanism (the degree to which the organisation is externally networked)</li><li>Peer pressure</li><li>External policies and incentives</li></ul>
Inner setting	<ul><li>Structural characteristics</li><li>Networks and communities</li><li>Culture</li><li>Implementation climate</li><li>Readiness for implementation</li></ul>
Characteristics of individuals	<ul><li>Knowledge and beliefs about the intervention</li><li>Self-efficacy</li><li>Individual stage of change</li><li>Individual identification with the organisation</li><li>Other personal attributes</li></ul>
Process of implementation	<ul><li>Planning</li><li>Engaging</li><li>Executing</li><li>Reflecting and evaluating</li></ul>

Source: After Damschroder et al. (2009).

and range of theories that could potentially be relevant. The TDF was further refined in 2012 (Cane et al., 2012) and proposes 14 theoretical domains of potential behavioural determinants; in other words, 14 key areas that may influence how people respond to the introduction of an evidence-based change. The TDF has been used to develop both qualitative and quantitative tools to measure behavioural responses at an individual or team level, for example, through individual interviews, surveys and focus group discussions. The domains and some exemplar questions are summarised in Table 3.2.

Our third example is the Knowledge to Action Framework, sometimes abbreviated to K2A. This framework was developed from a concept analysis of 31 planned action or change theories and models in the fields of health and social sciences, education and management (Graham and Tetroe, 2010). The review of these existing theories and models informed the development of a seven-phase cycle for translating knowledge into action (Table 3.3). The cycle encompasses both knowledge creation and knowledge application and recognises the need to adapt research evidence to take account of the local context and culture in which implementation takes place. Like the change theories it is based upon, K2A adopts a systems perspective, with a focus on how things can be implemented not at the level of individuals, but within complex social systems. Although K2A does not specify particular roles to guide or facilitate the action cycle, the need for strategies to facilitate implementation is noted within the description of the framework (Graham and Tetroe, 2010).

Other researchers have compared implementation frameworks and models, such as PAR-IHS, CFIR and K2A, to identify their relative strengths and weaknesses. For example, Tabak and colleagues reviewed 61 published models for dissemination and implementation research (Tabak et al., 2012). PARIHS was one of the frameworks included in the review and the authors' analysis was that PARIHS focused solely on implementation (not dissemination), provided a mid-range level of detail on the operational steps of implementation and lacked a focus on system and policy-related issues of implementation. A similar finding was reported in a systematic review of frameworks and taxonomies of factors that might prevent or enable improvements in healthcare professional practice (Flottorp et al., 2013). This review identified seven broad determinants of practice under the domain headings of: guideline factors; individual health professional factors; patient factors; professional interactions; incentives and resources; capacity for organisational change; social, political and legal factors. None of the 12 frameworks studied were seen to be completely comprehensive when compared against the seven domains. PARIHS was judged to be lacking a focus on individual health professional factors and social, political and legal factors.

Drawing together the evidence on users' experiences of applying PARIHS and comparison of PARIHS to other frameworks and models, a number of common themes begin to emerge, notably:

- a lack of focus on the individuals who have to implement the evidence (in whatever form that may be);
- a lack of focus on the wider, system level context in which implementation takes place, including policy, legal, social and political factors;
- a lack of operational detail on how to apply PARIHS in practice.

These findings have reinforced our own experiences of using PARIHS and have contributed to our thinking about a revised version of the framework, both in terms of the main

TABLE 3.2 The Theoretical Domains Framework (TDF)

Domain	Exemplar questions
Knowledge	• Is the recipient (individual/team) familiar with the guideline/evidence/innovation? • What do they think it says? • What do they think about the underlying evidence base?
Skills	• Do they know how to implement the intervention/s associated with the innovation? • How easy or difficult is it? • What skills does it require?
Social/professional role and identity	• Do they think undertaking the intervention/s in question is part of their role? • Are there any issues in relation to their peer group that influence how they can apply the evidence/innovation? • Are there any legal or ethical issues?
Beliefs about capabilities	• Do they feel confident to implement the changes associated with the innovation? • Have any problems been encountered?
Beliefs about consequences	• What are the consequences of implementing the innovation — likely costs, harms and benefits? • Do the perceived benefits outweigh the costs/harms?
Optimism	• What do they think will happen if they are not able to implement the innovation?
Intentions	• Do they intend to implement the innovation in practice? • Are any problems anticipated?
Memory, attention and decision processes	• How easy or difficult is it to apply the innovation in practice? • Are there situations where it is difficult? • What triggers the decision to practice in a particular way?
Environmental context and resources	• What factors inside and outside of the clinical environment affect the ability to implement the innovation? • Are there particular constraints that affect implementation?
Social influences	• Do other people that they work with influence their decision and/or ability to implement the innovation?
Emotions	• Do their own emotions and feelings affect implementation (e.g. worries or concerns about the innovation)? • Do patients' and families' emotions affect decision-making?
Goals	• Do they want to implement the innovation? • How important is it judged to be?
Behavioural regulation	• Are there things that encourage more consistent use of the innovation in practice?
Reinforcement	• Are there any personal or external incentives that might help to improve the uptake of the innovation?

Source: Adapted from Cane et al. (2012), Squires et al. (2013).

TABLE 3.3 Key features of the Knowledge to Action (K2A) framework

Phase of cycle	Contextual factors that need to be considered throughout the cycle
Identify the problem; identify, review and select knowledge	Nature of the evidence/knowledge: is it compelling and does it justify the innovation?
Adapt knowledge to local context	Attributes of the change/innovation: is it consistent with values, goals and needs?
Assess barriers and supports to knowledge use	Audience: various audiences that will be affected during implementation
Select, tailor, implement interventions	Context/culture: physical, social and organisational aspects of the implementation setting
Monitor knowledge use	Resources/support: are these sufficient?
Evaluate outcomes Sustain knowledge use	Implementation-related factors: strategies or factors to facilitate implementation

Source: Adapted from Graham and Tetroe (2010).

constructs and the need for a more explicit description of the facilitation roles and processes that are needed to operationalise it.

A more general observation in relation to the reviews that we have discussed concerns the terminology around implementation theories, frameworks and models which can be quite confusing. In some of the literature, 'theory' is used in a generic sense to incorporate models and frameworks for implementation. However, as we move through the remainder of the chapter, we will be using the term in a more discriminatory way. As such, when we talk about theory, we will be referring to an idea or set of ideas intended to represent facts or events in an explanatory or predictive way. By contrast, a conceptual framework aims to identify a set of variables and relationships that can be examined in order to understand a set of ideas or phenomena and a model is more prescriptive in that it specifies a particular set of actions or issues that need to be addressed.

When PARIHS was developed, it was presented as a conceptual framework that set out the key variables that were thought to influence successful implementation, namely evidence, context and facilitation (Kitson et al., 1998). As part of refining and developing the framework further, we examined the distinction between theories, frameworks and models (Kitson et al., 2008) and recognised that multiple theories could be consistent with PARIHS. The inductive way in which PARIHS was originally developed meant that the consideration of relevant theories was largely implicit in the original conceptualisation of the framework. However, through the concept analyses of the constructs of evidence (Rycroft-Malone et al., 2004), context (McCormack et al., 2002) and facilitation (Harvey et al., 2002), and the subsequent refinement and evaluation of PARIHS (Rycroft-Malone et al., 2002; Kitson et al., 2008), we began to consider theory more explicitly and develop greater clarity around theories that were consistent with the underlying assumptions of PARIHS. Furthermore, from our own experiences of applying PARIHS and working in the field of facilitation and implementation research, we have continued to develop our understanding of theories that have proved helpful in terms of thinking about, practising and researching the facilitation of evidence-based practice. Before moving on to describe our revisions to the PARIHS framework, we will briefly discuss some of the main theories that have contributed to our thinking.

Theories informing our understanding of implementation and facilitation

Just as there are multiple frameworks and models in the field of implementation and evidence-based practice, so too there are a range of theories that are relevant to this field of study, drawn from a wide range of disciplines. Our intention here is not to provide a detailed overview of these theories, but rather to point the reader in the direction of useful summaries and to high-light the key theories that have been influential in developing our own approach to facilitating implementation.

Our selection of which theories to include is essentially pragmatic; we have focused on theories that help to explain or predict what facilitation approaches need to take into account in relation to what is being implemented (the evidence or innovation), who is affected (the intended target groups for implementation) and where (the context). In each case we will briefly describe the main tenets of the theory and how and why it has contributed to our thinking. As noted, this is not intended to be an exhaustive discussion, but rather to give some background to the theories that we will draw upon in the following sections and chapters of the book as we present the revised i-PARIHS conceptual framework and the model of facili-tation that we are proposing to operationalise i-PARIHS. For more detailed information on the theoretical literature that pertains to implementation science, we would recommend the references listed in Box 3.1.

BOX 3.1   USEFUL READING ON THE ROLE OF THEORY IN IMPLEMENTATION

Eccles, M., Grimshaw, J., Walker, A., Johnston, M. & Pitts, N. 2005. Changing the behavior of healthcare professionals: the use of theory in promoting the uptake of research findings. *Journal of Clinical Epidemiology*, 58, 107–12.

Michie, S., Johnston, M., Abraham, C., Lawton, R., Parker, D. & Walker, A. 2005. Making psycho-logical theory useful for implementing evidence based practice: a consensus approach. *Quality and Safety Health Care*, 14, 26–33.

Estabrooks, C.A., Thompson, D.S., Lovely, J.J. & Hofmeyer, A. 2006. A guide to knowledge transla-tion theory. *Journal of Continuing Education in the Health Professions*, 26, 25–36.

Grol, R.P., Bosch, M.C., Hulscher, M.E., Eccles, M.P. & Wensing, M. 2007. Planning and studying improvement in patient care: the use of theoretical perspectives. *Milbank Quarterly*, 85, 93–138.

Rycroft-Malone, J. 2007. Theory and knowledge translation: setting some coordinates. *Nursing Research*, 56, S78–S85.

Michie, S., Van Stralen, M. & West, R. 2011. The behaviour change wheel: A new method for characterising and designing behaviour change interventions. *Implementation Science*, 6, 42.

Cane, J., O'Connor, D. & Michie, S. 2012. Validation of the theoretical domains framework for use in behaviour change and implementation research. *Implementation Science*, 7, 37.

Theories informing our views about evidence

From its early development, PARIHS adopted an eclectic view of evidence, informed by earlier reflections on the integration of deductive and inductive methods of knowledge generation (Kitson et al., 1996). So while the PARIHS framework was a response to the evidence-based healthcare movement, and specifically how to promote the uptake of research evidence in practice, we proposed that research was only one of the constituent elements of evidence that influenced practice. Consequently 'good' research evidence was a necessary but not sufficient component of strong evidence. Other dimensions of evidence, including clinical, patient and local experience and information were seen to be equally important (Rycroft-Malone et al., 2004).

This multi-dimensional view of evidence embraced different ways of 'knowing' and is informed by theories of problem-based, experiential and situated learning. The development of *problem-based learning* is credited to McMaster University in Canada, specifically in the design and delivery of its medical education programmes (Neville, 2009). This student-centred approach to learning focused on promoting learning through the experience of problem-solving in order to develop students' intrinsic motivation for learning and support the acquisition of self-directed learning and flexible knowledge. Similar to problem-based learning approaches, *experiential learning theory* emphasises learning from direct experience through reflection on doing (Kolb, 1984). Kolb proposed a reflective cycle of learning, moving from concrete experiences to reflective observation, abstract conceptualisation and active experimentation in the development of knowledge and skills. In a similar vein, *situated learning theory* highlights the importance of learning that takes place in the same context as which it is applied (Lave and Wenger, 1991).

What these various theories have in common is their focus on connecting knowledge with practice and experience and emphasising the importance of tacit knowledge (Polanyi, 1966). This is consistent with our conceptualisation of evidence within the original PARIHS framework, as something encompassing multiple sources of formal, explicit and experiential, tacit knowledge. Interestingly, the development of the evidence-based medicine movement also originated out of McMaster as an extension of the developments around problem-based learning, but with a specific focus on making sure that research evidence was consciously used to inform decision-making (Sackett et al., 1996). However, the application of evidence-based medicine has typically emphasised research as the primary source of evidence to inform practice, as exemplified by commonly used hierarchies of evidence which prioritise rigorous research evidence derived from systematic reviews of randomised controlled trials (OCEBM Levels of Evidence Working Group, 2014). The resultant effect has been to preference formal, explicit knowledge in the form of research and within this, to preference certain types of research.

As we have worked with PARIHS over the years and thought about the processes of implementation, we have also drawn more on *theories of innovation*, particularly the work of Everett Rogers and Andy Van de Ven, both of whom emphasise the involvement of end-users in knowledge creation and use. Rogers produced seminal work on the *diffusion of innovations* (Rogers, 1995), proposing that innovation was anything perceived as new by its audience and suggesting an alternative approach to conventional theories of change. Rather than focusing on encouraging or persuading people to change, diffusion of innovation theory looks at both the evolution of the innovation and the behaviour of individuals to achieve a better fit in terms of implementation. Thus innovation is not seen to be fixed or static, but something that is subject to re-invention and continuous improvement through involving intended users as active partners within its design and development. Rogers identified key features of an innovation that determine its likely adoption, suggesting that together the five factors listed below accounted for 49–87 per cent of the variation in adoption of new products (Rogers, 2003):

- Relative advantage
- Compatibility with existing values and practice
- Simplicity and ease of use
- Trialability
- Observable results.

Van de Ven is another researcher who has produced important insights into innovation (Van de Ven et al., 1999; Van de Ven, 2007). Reporting on the Minnesota Innovation Research Programme, Van de Ven and colleagues presented longitudinal field research on 14 different innovations over a period of 17 years (Van de Ven et al., 1999). A key finding was that the process of innovation was not sequential and orderly as previously described, but neither was it totally random and chaotic. Instead, a non-linear, dynamic system with diverging and converging cycles over time was observed, with enabling and constraining factors at different organisational levels acting to create convergence or divergence. Innovation was seen to be a collective, as opposed to individual, achievement and dependent on distributed knowledge. Attention to and investment in internal processes such as learning networks, leadership behaviours and cultural focus were seen to be important enablers of the innovation cycle. A key message emerging from this study was the need to 'go with the flow' of the innovation journey, not trying to control it but learning the best way to manoeuvre through the process.

In a subsequent body of work, Van de Ven proposed a theory of *engaged scholarship* (Van de Ven and Johnson, 2006; Van de Ven, 2007), which he described as a form of inquiry where researchers worked with intended users of research to deal with real-world, complex problems and co-create knowledge. Rather than seeing the theory–practice dilemma as a 'gap' requiring a knowledge transfer solution, Van de Ven proposed that it was actually a knowledge production problem that needed to be addressed by more engaged forms of scholarship.

Theories informing our views about the intended target groups for implementation

As the previous discussion of theories relating to evidence highlights, if we adopt an innovation perspective then the intended audience or target group is seen as part of the innovation process. This is consistent with the PARIHS conceptualisation of implementation, although originally the target groups for implementation were not specifically identified within the framework. Users and critics of PARIHS have highlighted the lack of focus on the recipients, in particular individuals, as a weakness of the framework.

In examining theories relating to the intended audience for implementation, some of these are contained within the innovation literature – not surprising since users are seen as a fundamental part of the *innovation process*. For example, Rogers highlighted the importance of understanding different groups within the intended audience for innovation and how they are likely to react, from innovators, early adopters and the early majority through to the late majority and laggards. In bringing different groups on board, emphasis was placed on the importance of peer-to-peer conversations and networks and the role of credible and trusted teachers and leaders (Rogers, 1995, 2003). In their review of the diffusion, dissemination and implementation of innovations in health service delivery and organisation, Greenhalgh and colleagues highlighted a number of key characteristics of the adopter, including their needs, motivations, values and goals, skills, learning style and social networks (Greenhalgh et al., 2004).

Similar themes relating to these adopter characteristics and behaviours are reflected in the previously described Theoretical Domains Framework (Michie et al., 2005; Cane et al., 2012), where motivation is considered alongside factors such as role and identity, goals, behavioural regulation, beliefs and capabilities and consequences. As discussed, this framework recognised and synthesised the vast number of theories that help to explain individual behavioural change. Within our analysis, we are particularly interested in theories of individual motivation and behaviour that link to the way in which knowledge is used in practice. One theory that we have found useful in this respect is the *theory of organisational readiness to change* (Weiner, 2009). Although described in terms of organisational readiness, the theory proposes that readiness depends upon collective behaviour change linked to two key factors, described as change commitment (in other words, do the intended targets want to change) and change efficacy (are they able to change). Determinants of change commitment and change efficacy are summarised in Table 3.4.

Other theories that we would suggest are useful in understanding how people respond to and influence implementation are those that look at the interactions and boundaries between different groups, for example, *communities of practice theory* and the *theory of sticky knowledge*. We also look at *boundary theory* and how boundaries can affect the ease with which new knowledge is translated and implemented.

Communities of practice theory was developed by Etienne Wenger, drawing on earlier ideas about situated learning that we discussed in the previous section (Lave and Wenger, 1991; Wenger, 1998). Communities of practice (COPs) are formed by people who share a common concern and engage in a process of collective learning about their joint interest. A COP is more than a group as it fulfils three distinguishing characteristics, namely: a shared domain of interest, joint activity and discussion and shared practice. As such, COPs are not limited by formal structures and can be formed across organisational and geographical boundaries, for example, involving people from the same professional group or with an interest in the same

TABLE 3.4 Determinants of change commitment and change efficacy

Change commitment	Change efficacy
• Underpinned by motivation theories	• Underpinned by social cognitive theory
• Perceived value of the proposed change in terms of whether it is needed, important or worthwhile	• Task demands (understanding what the change entails)
• Potential to generate improvement	• Resource availability (human, financial, material, informational)
• Resonance with core values	• Situation factors (time availability, internal politics, etc.)
• Visible support from respected colleagues, managers or leaders	

Source: After Weiner (2009).

clinical issue. COP theory has been applied quite widely within healthcare, particularly within studies of quality improvement and evidence-based practice, for example (Gabbay et al., 2003; Le May, 2009; Kislov et al., 2012). One finding that emerges from these studies is that COPs can be highly effective in terms of generating and sharing new knowledge among members; however, the boundaries they create around themselves can act to impede knowledge flow beyond the COP (Kislov, 2014).

This concept of boundaries links to Szulanski's *sticky knowledge theory* (Szulanski, 1996). Szulanski studied how best practice was shared and transferred within eight different companies and suggested that it was not motivational factors that acted as the main barriers. Rather, knowledge was seen to be sticky due to a combination of knowledge-related, recipient and contextual factors. In terms of the knowledge to be transferred, issues relating to ambiguity and irreducible uncertainty, linked to the tacit nature of knowledge and how it produced an effect, were seen to produce stickiness. A key recipient factor was described in terms of the absorptive capacity of the recipient, determined by their prior level of knowledge and their ability to make effective use of new knowledge. A third factor related to the nature of the relationship between the source and the recipient of the new knowledge, in terms of closeness and the ease of communication. Where this relationship was laborious and distant, the likelihood of sticky knowledge was increased. Based on these findings, Szulanski proposed that organisations need to focus on developing their learning capacity, fostering relationships and systematically understanding and communicating practice (Szulanski, 1996).

Carlile has provided further insights into the notion of *boundaries* and how they affect the way in which knowledge flows (Carlile, 2002, 2004). Through an ethnographic study in four different commercial sectors and adopting a perspective of 'knowledge in practice,' Carlile identified three different types of boundaries, which in order of complexity were described as syntactic, semantic and pragmatic boundaries. Syntactic boundaries existed where the individuals and teams involved in giving or receiving new knowledge experienced some differences in the language and terminology they used, but were able to reach a solution by finding a common syntax. A more complex boundary – a semantic boundary – arose when there were different interpretations of the knowledge. Hence there was a need to find a way of establishing and agreeing a common meaning. The most complex boundary was termed a pragmatic boundary, which was likely to exist where the new knowledge introduced a greater degree of novelty. Here more than a difference in language or meaning was encountered; knowledge was seen to be at stake and had to be negotiated across the boundary.

Building on this boundary theory, Carlile proposed that different strategies were required to address syntactic, semantic and pragmatic boundaries (Carlile, 2004). At a syntactic boundary, knowledge transfer strategies were seen to be sufficient, built around an agreed language and set of messages. At a semantic boundary, the emphasis needed to shift to a translational strategy to achieve a sense of collective meaning, whereas at a pragmatic boundary a more transformational approach was required to address the complex issues around the knowledge differences between different groups, for example, in relation to power, vested interests and politics.

Theories informing our views about the context of implementation

In terms of the context of implementation, the theories that have particularly influenced our thinking include those that deal with issues of organisational complexity and theories about how organisations learn and use new knowledge. To illustrate this, we will discuss *complexity, absorptive capacity* and *learning organisation* theories. We will also consider theories relating to *leadership* and *organisational culture*, which were recognised as important dimensions of context within the original PARIHS framework (McCormack et al., 2002) and highlighted by Van de Ven et al. (1999) as key enablers of innovation. Finally, we will look at theories that inform our understanding of *sustainability* and external influences on the context of implementation.

Complexity theory or complex adaptive systems is a collection of theories derived from multiple disciplines that involves the study of systems where individual units within the system can act in ways that are not totally predictable, but neither are they totally random. Plsek and Greenhalgh (2001) considered the application of complexity theory within healthcare and identified a number of its distinguishing characteristics, as summarised in Box 3.2. On the basis of such complexity, there is a need for organisations and the individuals within them to develop adaptive behaviours, rather than trying to fix problems and remove ambiguity or uncertainty. This requires attention to what Argyris and Schon (1996) described as double-loop or reflective learning and involves the application of approaches that combine knowledge and experience, consistent with the previously discussed theories of experiential learning.

BOX 3.2 DISTINGUISHING FEATURES OF COMPLEX ADAPTIVE SYSTEMS THEORY

- Fuzzy boundaries
- Fluid membership
- Self-organisation through simple, locally applied rules (e.g. mental models, instincts, constructs)
- Adapts behaviour over time
- Embedded in and interacts with other systems, leading to:

  - tension and paradox
  - emergent, novel behaviour
  - inherent non-linearity and unpredictability
  - patterns of behaviour

After Plsek and Greenhalgh (2001).

Learning organisation theory is again a collection of different theories that examine how organisations learn. Multiple theories are relevant here (for further reference see Easterby-Smith and Lyles, 2011); however, the term 'learning organisation' was coined by Senge (1990), referring to an organisation that actively transforms itself by facilitating the learning of its members. Five distinguishing features of learning organisations were proposed, namely: systems thinking; personal mastery (continual self-improvement of employees); mental models (culture); shared vision; and team learning. The focus was on encouraging organisations to move towards more organic and interconnected ways of thinking and operating, with an emphasis on fostering collectivity and communities.

Absorptive capacity theory derives from the study of strategic management and focuses on how organisations acquire, assimilate and apply new knowledge from the environment in order to innovate and achieve better performance outcomes (Cohen and Levinthal, 1990). A distinction is made between an organisation's potential and realised absorptive capacity, where potential capacity relates to the acquisition and assimilation of knowledge (which gives organisations the flexibility they need to adapt in rapidly changing environments) and realised capacity, which involves the transformation and exploitation of knowledge (Zahra and George, 2002). In order to identify, assimilate and apply new knowledge, and adapt to changing environments, organisations need to have absorptive capacities, which are based on relevant prior knowledge, and coordinating mechanisms to enhance formal and informal knowledge exchange (Harvey et al., 2009).

Multiple leadership theories are apparent in the literature, taking a range of different perspectives. These have been classified in various ways, for example, hierarchical versus distributed or shared leadership (McKee et al., 2013). Studies looking at the role of leadership in relation to improvement and innovation in healthcare (Van de Ven et al., 1999; Ovretveit, 2009; McKee et al., 2013) emphasise the importance of newer, *distributed theories of leadership*. Rather than focusing on what individuals in leadership roles do – as is the case with theories such as trait, transactional and transformational leadership – distributed leadership theory emphasises the collective, social process of leadership. Thus leadership operates at multiple levels, involves many different people and works through relationships, rather than individual action. This is consistent with the literature on leadership for evidence-based practice, which highlights the need for both formal and informal leaders, functioning in different roles at strategic and functional levels within the organisation (for example, Stetler et al., 2014).

Similar to leadership, *organisational culture* is an area where multiple different theories exist. These typically distinguish between seeing culture as something that an organisation possesses and culture as something that is synonymous with the organisation. Schein (2004) addresses this issue by suggesting three levels of culture within organisations, which he describes as artefacts, espoused values and shared basic assumptions. Artefacts and rituals are the most outwardly observable aspects of culture, in the form of organisational structure, processes, rules and rituals. Espoused values are manifest in the organisational strategy, philosophy and goals; in turn, these are underpinned by tacit, taken-for-granted beliefs, which are seen to be the ultimate source of values, decision-making and action within the organisation. Understanding these more hidden, shared assumptions is essential to fully comprehend the culture of the organisation.

Sustainability is concerned with embedding the changes introduced by an innovation, such that they become the normal way of working. Again, various theories aim to explain how and why sustainability can be achieved, in order that the improvements made do not evaporate or decay. One theory that has been applied quite widely in healthcare is *normalisation process theory* (May et al., 2009; McEvoy et al., 2014), described as an action theory to enable implementation and integration of innovations in practice. The theory proposes four constructs that represent the generative mechanisms required to routinely embed innovations, namely: coherence, cognitive participation, collective action and reflexive monitoring (May and Finch, 2009). A potential source of tension between the routine embedding of change and creating organisational inertia is recognised in the literature, as the act of normalising could be seen to run counter to the need for individuals, teams and organisations to be constantly adapting and changing. In order to address this so-called 'dilemma of sustainability', Buchanan et al. (2007) propose a processual model of sustainability in context. This recognises the multiple factors that impact on sustainability and the need to balance maintaining the gains with further innovation and development over time.

A final set of theories relevant to the study of context are those that govern the external environment of the healthcare system, for example, *theories of regulation, market economy, financial incentives and contracting*. A summary of some of the main political and economic theories of interest is provided by Grol et al. (2007). Unlike the theories we have described relating to the innovation, the recipients and the internal context, where the facilitator can apply the ideas contained within the various theories to guide the implementation process, the immediate relevance of theories relating to the external context may be less direct. The important thing is to be aware of and understand the potential influence of external factors when planning and facilitating implementation, as we will discuss further in the following chapter.

Common themes running through these theories

From this brief overview of theories, a number of common themes are apparent, which to a large extent converge across the dimensions of evidence, recipients and context. Generally, these theories reinforce the complex, dynamic and non-linear nature of implementation and emphasise the importance of collective, experiential learning at the level of individuals, teams and organisations. What is also apparent is the interrelationship between aspects of the innovation, the recipients and the context. Table 3.5 summarises the key themes that emerge from theories relating to the 'what', 'who' and 'where' of implementation and implications for the 'how' issues of implementation. We then move on to outline which theories of facilitation have been influential in our analysis and interpretation of the themes highlighted in Table 3.5.

Theories informing our views about facilitation

As Table 3.5 highlights, the themes identified from our theoretical analysis have important implications for the way in which the process of implementation is approached. Broadly speaking, these highlight the need for processes that recognise and adapt to the dynamic and situation-specific nature of implementation, with an emphasis on building relationships, learning and flexibility. We believe that the concept of facilitation – with its focus on enabling others to act – provides an ideal way in which to embrace such principles in a flexible and responsive way. In developing the model of facilitation that we describe in subsequent chapters of the book, we have drawn from a number of key theorists, notably Carl Rogers, John Heron and W. Edwards Deming.

Carl Rogers was a psychologist and influential member of the humanist approach to psychology, essentially focused on promoting more person-centred approaches. This same philosophy was subsequently applied within the field of education, where Rogers argued for a shift in focus from teaching to the facilitation of learning (Rogers, 1969). This required teachers to accept the role of mentors and guides, rather than the imparters of knowledge. In turn, this implied a need to recognise the different learning styles of students, to build on prior experience and make learning relevant, to create an atmosphere of trust and openness and encourage open-mindedness.

John Heron similarly comes from a humanist perspective, facilitating approaches to cooperative inquiry within the fields of counselling, personal and professional development (Heron, 1989). Heron proposed six distinct modes of facilitator intervention, which he described as planning, structuring, (creating) meaning, (addressing) feeling, valuing and confronting.

TABLE 3.5 Themes emerging from key elements of implementation theory

Focus of implementation	Themes identified from theoretical analysis
WHAT is being implemented? Characteristics of the evidence, knowledge or innovation	• Broad definitions of evidence, linked to wider literature on innovation and knowledge generation and application • Embedded and emergent; influence and contribution of tacit knowledge • Importance of experiential and situated learning • Value of co-production
WHO is being targeted? Characteristics of the target groups for implementation	• Recognition of 'want to' and 'can do' factors (motivation and capability/capacity) • Importance of collectivity and learning within communities • Different responses to innovation and change • Different learning styles • Existence of boundaries between different groups/communities • Increasingly complex boundaries as innovation increases in novelty • Influence of social networks
WHERE? Characteristics of the setting in which implementation takes place	• Organisations as complex, adaptive systems • Emphasis on learning at the individual, team and organisational level • Influence of culture and mental models • Influence of prior knowledge and experience • Importance of collaboration, coordination and networks for knowledge exchange
HOW? Implications for the process of implementation	• Distributed learning – through teams and networks • Importance of flexibility and adaptability • Tailoring approaches to different needs and responses • Reflective learning • Credible and trusted leaders and teachers • Distributed/shared leadership • Building relationships • Understanding and communicating practices

These were the key areas where facilitators needed to focus their attention in order to enable the achievement of goals (for example, through structuring and planning the experience) and manage the process effectively (for example, by supporting and valuing individuals, confronting sources of resistance, developing a shared meaning and addressing group feelings). Throughout the facilitation encounter, Heron suggested that the facilitator could adopt different levels of control, ranging from a directive through a cooperative to a totally non-directive approach, depending on the specific needs of the group or situation.

Rogers' and Heron's perspectives on facilitation provide a general framing of our approach, namely one that is focused on enabling, guiding and supporting, rather than persuading, telling or instructing. We have combined these general principles with improvement theory and methods in order to operationalise a model of facilitation for evidence-based practice. This involves building on our earlier work in the field of quality improvement, with an emphasis on participative and locally owned approaches to auditing and improving the quality of care (as described in Chapter 2), alongside the wider literature on quality management and continuous quality improvement. Of particular note is the work of W. Edwards Deming and his description of the *system of profound knowledge* (Deming, 2000). Deming was an engineer and statistician who devoted a large part of his life to practising, learning and writing about quality management. This culminated in the system of profound knowledge, which he presented as a management philosophy for organisations to continuously thrive and improve. The system of profound knowledge comprises four interrelated components, defined as: appreciation of a system (understanding the whole process and the interactions and interdependencies within the system); understanding variation (distinguishing between different types of variation through the analysis of data and application of statistical processes); a theory of knowledge (testing theories and hunches against data through the use of Plan–Do–Study–Act cycles); and knowledge of psychology (understanding people and the need to develop trust, relationships and interdependence).

Although we do not explicitly apply Deming's system of profound knowledge within the model of facilitation we present in Chapter 4, we draw on the principles embodied within it, as it touches on many of the themes that we identified in Table 3.5. Similarly, we will make links to other relevant theories that help to inform and operationalise facilitation as we move through subsequent chapters of the book. We turn now to presenting the revised version of the PARIHS framework, based on the integration of theoretical, empirical and experiential evidence.

Introducing the i-PARIHS framework

As the discussion in the chapter to date illustrates, there are a number of reasons for re-visiting the original PARIHS framework before we set out a facilitation model for its operationalisation. These include:

- reviews of the framework that suggest its core constructs fail to address the intended targets for implementation and the wider external context;
- empirical research that highlights the influential role of individuals in determining the processes and outcomes of implementation;
- a synthesis of key theories related to implementing evidence, new knowledge and innovation in practice.

From our analysis and synthesis of this evidence, we think that the constructs of the PARIHS framework need to be revised, as does the relationship of facilitation to the other constructs. In our original conceptualisation of PARIHS, we proposed that successful implementation was a function of the interplay between evidence, context and facilitation. This was expressed as a simple equation (Box 3.3), although as critics rightly pointed out, we did not clearly define what we meant by 'successful implementation' (Helfrich et al., 2010; Stetler et al., 2011). In our revised, i-PARIHS framework, we are suggesting that successful implementation results from the facilitation of an innovation with the recipients in their (inner and outer) context (Box 3.4). Consequently, the core constructs within i-PARIHS are facilitation, innovation, recipients and context, with facilitation as the active element assessing, aligning and integrating the other three constructs. Successful implementation is defined on a number of levels, reflecting the multi-dimensional focus on the innovation, the recipients and the context. The rationale for the proposed changes and the implications in terms of applying the framework are summarised below.

BOX 3.3   'SUCCESSFUL IMPLEMENTATION' IN THE ORIGINAL PARIHS FRAMEWORK

$$SI = f(E,C,F)$$

- SI = Successful implementation
- f = Function (of)
- E = Evidence
- C = Context
- F = Facilitation

BOX 3.4   'SUCCESSFUL IMPLEMENTATION' IN THE I-PARIHS FRAMEWORK

$$SI = Fac^n(I + R + C)$$

- SI = Successful implementation:
    - Achievement of agreed implementation/project goals
    - The uptake and embedding of the innovation in practice
    - Individuals, teams and stakeholders are engaged, motivated and 'own' the innovation
    - Variation related to context is minimised across implementation settings

- Fac^n = Facilitation
- I = Innovation
- R = Recipients (individual and collective)
- C = Context (inner and outer)

The innovation construct

We have extended the concept of evidence to the broader notion of innovation. This is for a number of reasons. First, the broad definition of evidence that we originally proposed within PARIHS meant that people using the framework approached implementation from different starting points. In some cases, this involved implementing an established 'piece' of evidence such as a systematic review or a clinical guideline – in line with more conventional models of evidence-based practice. However, in other cases the starting point was a local issue identified through a clinical audit, observations of care or patient feedback. As such, the project resembled a typical service improvement project, with evidence generated or gathered as part of the initial stages of scoping the problem and establishing goals for improvement. Second, given this broad interpretation of evidence, and our reading of the literature, we believe there is benefit to be gained from thinking more widely about knowledge and how knowledge is generated, mobilised and exchanged within and between organisations. This position recognises the role of both explicit and tacit knowledge in informing decision-making and practice at a clinical and organisational level. Third, our review of relevant theories has led us into the literature outside the conventional fields of evidence-based practice and healthcare, particularly to theories of innovation and knowledge management. This provides useful insights which we think help to further our understanding of implementation, particularly in terms of the interconnections between knowledge and practice (for example, situated and experiential learning, co-creation of knowledge) and understanding the characteristics of knowledge that enhance or inhibit its uptake.

Consequently, we are proposing 'innovation' as a central construct within the i-PARIHS framework, but with an explicit focus on sourcing and applying available research evidence to inform the innovation. Box 3.5 summarises key features that need to be considered within the innovation construct.

BOX 3.5 CHARACTERISTICS OF THE INNOVATION TO BE CONSIDERED IN IMPLEMENTATION

- Underlying knowledge sources
- Clarity
- Degree of fit with existing practice and values (compatibility or contestability)
- Degree of novelty
- Useability
- Relative advantage
- Trialability
- Observable results

The recipient construct

This is a new construct that we have added to i-PARIHS, reflecting the views of users and reviewers, namely that the original PARIHS framework paid insufficient attention to the intended targets for implementation. This position is supported by the theoretical literature which highlights the influence that recipient characteristics can have on the processes and outcomes of implementation. Although some empirical evidence suggests that individuals should be represented as an additional construct within PARIHS (for example, Rycroft-Malone et al., 2013), we consider recipients at both individual and team level. This reflects the role that individual leaders can play in supporting or resisting innovation. However, the theoretical literature also highlights the importance of working through teams, especially in terms of fostering learning and relationships, for example, through COPs. Equally, it is important to be cognisant of the boundaries that can exist between groups or teams and the potential barriers these can present during implementation. Box 3.6 identifies key characteristics of the recipients (both individual and team) that are important to take into account.

BOX 3.6 CHARACTERISTICS OF THE RECIPIENTS TO BE CONSIDERED IN IMPLEMENTATION

- Motivation
- Values and beliefs

- Goals
- Skills and knowledge
- Time, resources and support
- Local opinion leaders
- Collaboration and teamwork
- Existing networks
- Learning environment
- Power and authority
- Presence of boundaries

The context construct

Context remains as a core construct within i-PARIHS, but with a clearer recognition of both the inner and outer context. Inner context includes both the immediate setting for implementation, whether that is a hospital ward or department, a primary care clinic or general practice office, and the organisation in which that unit or department is located. Outer context refers to the wider health system in which the organisation is based and the policies, regulatory frameworks and political environment that govern the way in which the health system functions. Within each of these levels of context, which can be thought of in terms of micro, meso and macro levels, specific factors will be important, as presented in Table 3.6. These factors are influenced by a number of the theories previously discussed, for example, complexity theory, absorptive capacity and organisational learning.

The facilitation construct

As with the original PARIHS framework, facilitation remains a core construct within i-PARIHS. However, we emphasise facilitation as the active ingredient within i-PARIHS by positioning it differently in relation to the constructs of innovation, recipients and context (see Box 3.4). Rather than seeing facilitation as one of the three constructs that interplay to determine the outcomes of implementation, we conceptualise facilitation as the construct that activates implementation through assessing and responding to characteristics of the innovation

TABLE 3.6 Characteristics of the context to be considered in implementation

Inner context: local level	Inner context: organisational level	Outer context
• Formal and informal leadership support • Culture • Past experience of innovation and change • Mechanisms for embedding change • Evaluation and feedback processes	• Organisational priorities • Leadership and senior management support • Culture • Structure and systems • History of innovation and change • Absorptive capacity • Learning networks	• Policy drivers and priorities • Incentives and mandates • Regulatory frameworks • Environmental (in)stability • Inter-organisational networks and relationships

and the recipients within their contextual setting. This requires a role (the facilitator) and a set of strategies and actions (the facilitation process) to enable implementation. In Chapter 4, we will describe the model of facilitation that we are proposing to operationalise i-PARIHS. This builds on the theories that we have discussed, with an emphasis on both identifying and achieving goals for implementation, through the application of improvement methods and processes, and enabling the process of implementation, by working through teams and facilitating learning and development.

Summary

In this chapter, we have attempted to pull together a diverse set of empirical, experiential and theoretical literature that has informed the ongoing refinement of the PARIHS framework, resulting in the presentation of what we now describe as the integrated-PARIHS framework. This framework underpins the facilitation model that we present in the next chapter. It remains a work in progress as we continue to build our knowledge and experience within the field of implementation and facilitation. The theories that we have presented are an introduction to a vast repository of literature from a wide range of disciplines. As facilitators become more experienced in the role, this is likely to be an area that they will want to explore and develop further. This is something that we will return to as we discuss the facilitator's journey and application of the facilitation model in Chapters 5, 6 and 7.

References

Argyris, C. & Schon, D.A. 1996. *Organizational Learning II: Theory, Method and Practice*. Reading, MA: Addison-Wesley.

Buchanan, D., Fitzgerald, L. & Ketley, D. 2007. *The Sustainability and Spread of Organizational Change*. Abingdon, UK: Routledge.

Cane, J., O'Connor, D. & Michie, S. 2012. Validation of the theoretical domains framework for use in behaviour change and implementation research. *Implementation Science*, 7, 37.

Carlile, P.R. 2002. A pragmatic view of knowledge and boundaries: boundary objects in new product development. *Organization Science*, 13, 442–55.

Carlile, P.R. 2004. Transferring, translating, and transforming: an integrative framework for managing knowledge across boundaries. *Organization Science*, 15, 555–68.

Cohen, W.M. & Levinthal, D.A. 1990. Absorptive capacity: a new perspective on learning and innovation. *Administrative Science Quarterly*, 35, 128–52.

Damschroder, L., Aron, D., Keith, R., Kirsh, S., Alexander, J. & Lowery, J. 2009. Fostering implementation of health services research findings into practice: a consolidated framework for advancing implementation science. *Implementation Science*, 4, 50.

Deming, W.E. 2000. *Out of the Crisis*. Cambridge, MA: MIT Press.

Easterby-Smith, M. & Lyles, M. 2011. *Handbook of Organizational Learning and Knowledge Management* (2nd edn). Chichester: John Wiley & Sons.

Flottorp, S., Oxman, A., Krause, J., Musila, N., Wensing, M., Godycki-Cwirko, M., Baker, R. & Eccles, M. 2013. A checklist for identifying determinants of practice: A systematic review and synthesis of frameworks and taxonomies of factors that prevent or enable improvements in healthcare professional practice. *Implementation Science*, 8, 35.

Gabbay, J., Le May, A., Jefferson, H., Webb, D., Lovelock, R., Powell, J. & Lathlean, J. 2003. A case study of knowledge management in multiagency consumer-informed 'communities of practice': implications for evidence-based policy development in health and social services. *Health*, 7, 283–310.

Graham, I. & Tetroe, J.M. 2010. The Knowledge to Action Framework. In: Rycroft-Malone, J. & Bucknall, T. (eds.) *Models and Frameworks for Implementing Evidence-Based Practice: Linking Evidence to Action.* Chichester: Wiley-Blackwell.

Greenhalgh, T., Robert, G., Macfarlane, F., Bate, P. & Kyriakidou, O. 2004. Diffusion of innovations in service organizations: systematic review and recommendations. *Milbank Quarterly*, 82, 581–629.

Grol, R., Bosch, M., Hulscher, M., Eccles, M. & Wensing, M. 2007. Planning and studying improvement in patient care: the use of theoretical perspectives. *Milbank Quarterly*, 85, 93–138.

Harvey, G., Loftus-Hills, A., Rycroft-Malone, J., Titchen, A., Kitson, A., McCormack, B. & Seers, K. 2002. Getting evidence into practice: the role and function of facilitation. *Journal of Advanced Nursing*, 37, 577–88.

Harvey, G., Skelcher, C., Spencer, E., Jas, P. & Walshe, K. 2009. Absorptive capacity in a non-market environment. *Public Management Review*, 12, 77–97.

Helfrich, C., Damschroder, L., Hagedorn, H., Daggett, G., Sahay, A., Ritchie, M., et al. 2010. A critical synthesis of literature on the promoting action on research implementation in health services (PARIHS) framework. *Implementation Science*, 5, 82.

Heron, J. 1989. *The Facilitator's Handbook.* London: Kogan Page.

Kislov, R. 2014. Boundary discontinuity in a constellation of interconnected practices. *Public Administration*, 92, 307–23.

Kislov, R., Walshe, K. & Harvey, G. 2012. Managing boundaries in primary care service improvement: a developmental approach to communities of practice. *Implementation Science*, 7, 97.

Kitson, A., Ahmed, L.B., Harvey, G., Seers, K. & Thompson, D.R. 1996. From research to practice: one organizational model for promoting research-based practice. *Journal of Advanced Nursing*, 23, 430–40.

Kitson, A., Harvey, G. & McCormack, B. 1998. Enabling the implementation of evidence based practice: a conceptual framework. *Quality in Health Care*, 7, 149–59.

Kitson, A., Rycroft-Malone, J., Harvey, G., McCormack, B., Seers, K. & Titchen, A. 2008. Evaluating the successful implementation of evidence into practice using the PARIHS framework: theoretical and practical challenges (2008). *Implementation Science*, 3, 1.

Kolb, D. 1984. *Experiential Learning: Experience as the Source of Learning and Development.* Englewood Cliffs, NJ: Prentice Hall.

Lave, J. & Wenger, E. 1991. *Situated Learning. Legitimate Peripheral Participation.* Cambridge, UK: University of Cambridge Press.

Le May, A. 2009. *Communities of Practice in Health and Social Care.* Oxford: Wiley-Blackwell.

May, C. & Finch, T. 2009. Implementation, embedding, and integration: an outline of Normalization Process Theory. *Sociology*, 43, 535–54.

May, C., Mair, F., Finch, T., Macfarlane, A., Dowrick, C., Treweek, S., et al. 2009. Development of a theory of implementation and integration: Normalization Process Theory. *Implementation Science*, 4, 29.

McCormack, B., Kitson, A., Harvey, G., Rycroft-Malone, J., Titchen, A. & Seers, K. 2002. Getting evidence into practice: the meaning of 'context'. *Journal of Advanced Nursing*, 38, 94–104.

McEvoy, R., Ballini, L., Maltoni, S., O'Donnell, C., Mair, F. & Macfarlane, A. 2014. A qualitative systematic review of studies using the normalization process theory to research implementation processes. *Implementation Science*, 9, 2.

McKee, L., Charles, K., Dixon-Woods, M., Willars, J. & Martin, G. 2013. 'New' and distributed leadership in quality and safety in health care, or 'old' and hierarchical? An interview study with strategic stakeholders. *Journal of Health Services Research & Policy*, 18, 11–19.

Michie, S., Johnston, M., Abraham, C., Lawton, R., Parker, D. & Walker, A. 2005. Making psychological theory useful for implementing evidence based practice: a consensus approach. *Quality and Safety in Health Care*, 14, 26–33.

Neville, A.J. 2009. Problem-based learning and medical education forty years on. *Medical Principles and Practice*, 18, 1–9.

OCEBM Levels of Evidence Working Group 2014. *The Oxford Levels of Evidence 2* [Online]. Available: http://www.cebm.net/index.aspx?o=5653 [accessed 31 August 2014]

Ovretveit, J. 2009. *Evidence: Leading Improvement Effectively*. London: The Health Foundation.

Plsek, P.E. & Greenhalgh, T. 2001. The challenge of complexity in health care. *British Medical Journal*, 323, 625–28.

Polanyi, M. 1966. *The Tacit Dimension*. Chicago: University of Chicago Press.

Rogers, C.R. 1969. *Freedom to Learn – A View of What Education Might Become*. Columbus, OH: Charles Merrill.

Rogers, E.M. 1995. *Diffusion of Innovations* (4th edn). New York: Free Press.

Rogers, E.M. 2003. *Diffusion of Innovations* (5th edn). New York: Free Press.

Rycroft-Malone, J. & Bucknall, T. 2010. *Models and Frameworks for Implementing Evidence-Based Practice: Linking Evidence to Action*. Chichester: Wiley-Blackwell.

Rycroft-Malone, J., Kitson, A., Harvey, G., McCormack, B., Seers, K., Titchen, A. & Estabrooks, C. 2002. Ingredients for change: revisiting a conceptual framework. *Quality and Safety in Health Care*, 11, 174–80.

Rycroft-Malone, J., Seers, K., Titchen, A., Harvey, G., Kitson, A. & McCormack, B. 2004. What counts as evidence in evidence-based practice? *Journal of Advanced Nursing*, 47, 81–90.

Rycroft-Malone, J., Seers, K., Crichton, N., Chandler, J., Hawkes, C., Allen, C., Bullock, I. & Strunin, L. 2012. A pragmatic cluster randomised trial evaluating three implementation interventions. *Implementation Science*, 7, 80.

Rycroft-Malone, J., Seers, K., Chandler, J., Hawkes, C., Crichton, N., Allen, C., Bullock, I. & Strunin, L. 2013. The role of evidence, context, and facilitation in an implementation trial: implications for the development of the PARIHS framework. *Implementation Science*, 8, 28.

Sackett, D.L., Rosenberg, W.M., Gray, J.A., Haynes, R.B. & Richardson, W.S. 1996. Evidence based medicine: what it is and what it isn't. *British Medical Journal*, 312, 71-2.

Schein, E.H. 2004. *Organizational Culture and Leadership*. San Francisco, CA: Jossey-Bass.

Senge, P.M. 1990. *The Fifth Discipline: The Art and Practice of the Learning Organization*. New York: Doubleday.

Squires, J., Suh, K., Linklater, S., Bruce, N., Gartke, K., Graham, I., et al. 2013. Improving physician hand hygiene compliance using behavioural theories: a study protocol. *Implementation Science*, 8, 16.

Stetler, C., Damschroder, L., Helfrich, C. & Hagedorn, H. 2011. A guide for applying a revised version of the PARIHS framework for implementation. *Implementation Science*, 6, 99.

Stetler, C.B., Ritchie, J.A., Rycroft-Malone, J. & Charns, M.P. 2014. Leadership for evidence-based practice: strategic and functional behaviors for institutionalizing EBP. *Worldviews on Evidence-Based Nursing*, 11, 219–26.

Szulanski, G. 1996. Exploring internal stickiness: impediments to the transfer of best practice within the firm. *Strategic Management Journal*, 17, 27–43.

Tabak, R.G., Khoong, E.C., Chambers, D.A. & Brownson, R.C. 2012. Bridging research and practice. *American Journal of Preventive Medicine*, 43, 337–50.

Van de Ven, A.H. 2007. *Engaged Scholarship: A Guide to Organizational and Social Research*. Oxford: Oxford University Press.

Van de Ven, A.H. & Johnson, P.E. 2006. Knowledge for theory and practice. *Academy of Management Review*, 31, 802–21.

Van de Ven, A.H., Pollet, D., Garud, R. & Venkataraman, S. 1999. *The Innovation Journey*. New York: Oxford University Press.

Weiner, B. 2009. A theory of organizational readiness for change. *Implementation Science*, 4, 67.

Wenger, E. 1998. *Communities of Practice: Learning, Meaning and Identity*. Cambridge, UK: Cambridge University Press.

Zahra, S.A. & George, G. 2002. Absorptive capacity: a review, reconceptualization, and extension. *Academy of Management Review*, 27, 185–203.

4

A MODEL OF FACILITATION FOR EVIDENCE-BASED PRACTICE

Gill Harvey and Alison Kitson

Introduction

In this chapter we outline our working model of facilitation to operationalise the i-PARIHS framework and support evidence-based innovation in practice. As with any model, the intention is to provide more detailed guidance on how to apply the i-PARIHS framework, which we have suggested is through the process of facilitation (Box 4.1). Facilitation is positioned as the active ingredient in i-PARIHS, with one or more individuals in the designated role of facilitators, helping to navigate individuals and teams through the complex change processes involved and the contextual challenges they may encounter. This requires a sound understanding of the nature of the innovation to be introduced (the focus and content of the implementation process), the individuals and teams that have to enact the change (the recipients) and the environment in which they work (the local, organisational and health system context). As we described in the previous chapter, this essentially involves thinking about *what* is to be implemented, *who* with and *where*. Facilitation provides the '*how*' component of implementation.

BOX 4.1   FACILITATION AS THE ACTIVE INGREDIENT IN THE i-PARIHS FRAMEWORK

$$SI = Fac^n(I + R + C)$$

- SI = Successful implementation

  - Achievement of agreed implementation/project goals
  - The uptake and embedding of the innovation in practice
  - Individuals, teams and stakeholders are engaged, motivated and 'own' the innovation
  - Variation related to context is minimised across implementation settings

- Fac^n = Facilitation
- I = Innovation
- R = Recipients (individual and collective)
- C = Context (inner and outer)

As we outline the facilitation model, we will discuss important considerations from a facilitation perspective in relation to understanding and assessing each of the dimensions of innovation, recipients and context. We also indicate the type of activities that a facilitator might engage in to support meaningful action relating to the innovation, the recipients and the different levels of context. By the end of the chapter, our aim is to have presented the building blocks of a model that can be used in practice to plan and facilitate an implementation project. In Chapter 6, we will then illustrate the application of this facilitation model with a detailed description of the steps and processes involved in setting up and running an implementation project in practice.

Before beginning the detailed description of the model, there are a few important points to make, which the reader should bear in mind while working their way through the chapter:

1. A facilitator is rarely a lone agent, particularly when the implementation projects in question are large or wide-scale in focus. Although we refer to the facilitator in the singular, in practice they are likely to be part of a bigger facilitation team. Indeed, this is a desirable situation as we will explore when we consider different facilitator roles in Chapters 5 and 7. Within a team-based facilitation structure, different members of the team will take particular responsibility for some of the activities outlined below.
2. In some cases, the facilitation responsibility may be combined with another role, such as a clinical leader, practice development nurse, quality improvement coordinator or a clinical specialist liaison role. The specific label of 'facilitator' is not important; the key point is that the individuals function as facilitators in that they actively use facilitation methods and processes to enable and support implementation.
3. In practice the process of facilitation is fluid and interactive. Any attempt to describe it in the way we are doing runs the risk of making it appear more logical and sequential than what actually happens in the real world. Although we distinguish between discrete aspects of implementation (the innovation, the recipients and context), in reality the boundaries between these may be blurred; so, for example, activities relating to the recipients are likely to impinge upon issues relating to the local context. This is something we will explore further as we move through the chapter.
4. For many people, their first steps into facilitation are a new encounter and much of the learning about the role and the facilitation process takes place 'on the job'. Part of the purpose of this book is to try to make the process of facilitation more explicit and to describe the types of knowledge and skills that a facilitator needs to develop to be effective in the role. However, we recognise that seeing the whole picture in the way we set out the model in this chapter may be a bit overwhelming – and not a reasonable expectation for novice facilitators to be able to take on. In subsequent chapters, we will focus in more detail on the process of getting started in facilitation and how to build the necessary portfolio of knowledge and skills to address the multiple elements contained within the model.

Figure 4.1 illustrates how we see the facilitation process in relation to implementing a piece of evidence or a particular service change. In i-PARIHS, we use the collective term 'innovation' to describe the focus or content of the implementation effort. As the diagram suggests,

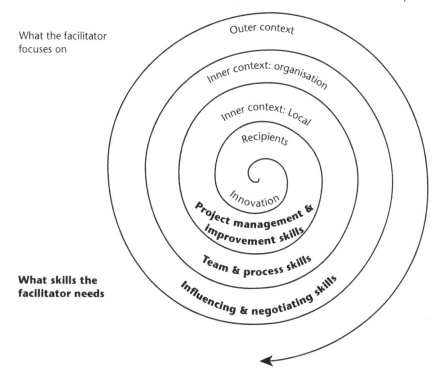

What the facilitator
focuses on

Outer context

Inner context: organisation

Inner context: Local

Recipients

Innovation

Project management &
improvement skills

Team & process skills

Influencing & negotiating skills

**What skills the
facilitator needs**

FIGURE 4.1 Levels of facilitation focus and skills

the facilitation process starts with a focus on the innovation in terms of thinking about planned and coordinated actions for implementation (Greenhalgh et al., 2004). However, in line with the assumptions of i-PARIHS, implementation involves a complex, multi-faceted process, with multiple interactions between the innovation to be implemented and the context within which implementation occurs. Within that context many different 'actors' are present at different levels of the health system, including individual patients and staff, teams, leaders, managers and policy-makers within the organisation and the wider health system. Consequently, 'what works' in terms of implementation in one setting may not work the same way in a different setting, meaning that the implementation process is not predictable. From a facilitation perspective, a useful way of understanding the interactive nature of implementation is to see the innovation as something that is nested in multiple levels from a micro, meso and macro organisational perspective – levels that are likely to be separated by professional, physical, cultural and political boundaries. Integrating evidence from the theories presented in the preceding chapter of the book with the elements of the i-PARIHS framework, the model specifies what the facilitator needs to focus on and what they need to do at each of the different levels. This is summarised in Figure 4.2 and each level – the innovation, the recipients, the inner and outer context – is outlined in more detail below, culminating in a series of reflective questions that the facilitator can use to navigate the different levels of implementation.

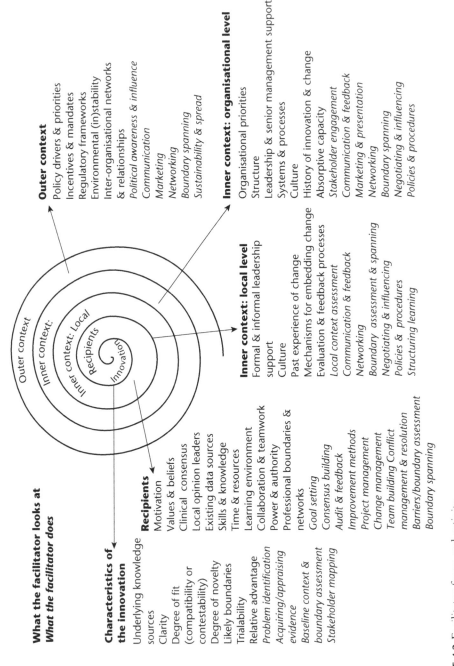

FIGURE 4.2 Facilitator focus and activity

The innovation

At the outset of the implementation process, the facilitator needs to give some thought to 'what' they are facilitating. Is it the implementation of an existing evidence product such as a clinical guideline or systematic review? If so, who developed the guideline and when was it published? Is it from a credible source that will be respected by the individuals and teams that the facilitator is working with and will it be perceived as timely and up to date? By contrast, if implementation is focused on a service change or improvement, questions that the facilitator might want to consider include: Who or what is driving the proposed change and why? What is the nature of the underlying problem that the proposed change is trying to address? Is there evidence to support the change in terms of clinical and cost-effectiveness? This is likely to involve the facilitator working with the individuals and teams concerned to clearly define the problem or the area for improvement, then sourcing and appraising available evidence to inform the change process and presenting this in a way that is accessible and understandable to key stakeholders.

To summarise, an important first step for the facilitator is exploring, examining and building an understanding about what the implementation effort is focused on: What is proposed and why? What evidence underpins the proposed implementation project? How credible and trustworthy is that evidence? However, establishing clarity about what is to be implemented does not equate to gaining agreement on the proposed implementation. This leads us to the next important consideration for the facilitator: What is the degree of fit between the innovation, the proposed change and the local setting? Here the facilitator needs to give thought to issues such as who is likely to be affected by the innovation and in what way? And, most importantly, how much consensus – or disagreement – is there likely to be? So in the case of a clinical guideline, will the different groups involved (professional groups, managers, patients) receive and respond to the evidence contained in the guideline in the same way? The literature on implementing evidence into practice illustrates very clearly that rigorous and robust research evidence is rarely enough to guarantee its uptake into practice; rather evidence is typically subject to negotiation, contestation and adaptation before it becomes implemented (Ferlie et al, 2000; Dopson and Fitzgerald, 2005).

In the original PARIHS framework, we mapped out the multi-dimensional nature of evidence, encompassing research, clinical, patient and local experience (see Chapter 2), and suggested that the more these are aligned the greater the likelihood of successfully implementing evidence into practice. There are also useful pointers in the literature on the diffusion of innovations (for example, Rogers, 1995; Greenhalgh et al, 2004) in terms of issues to think about relating to the actual innovation or change. For example, what, if any, advantage does the new evidence or innovation offer compared to the current way of doing things? And will all those affected perceive this in the same way? This is an important consideration in healthcare where much of the research evidence that underpins new interventions and systematic reviews addresses questions of effectiveness. In other words, does this intervention X produce outcomes Y? And is it more (clinically and/or cost) effective than intervention Z? These are valid and important questions; however, what matters to a patient may be more to do with the acceptability or accessibility of a proposed treatment intervention. Or at an organisational level, a senior manager might have to make decisions about multiple pieces of evidence and balance effectiveness with affordability and equity across the service as a whole. The innovation literature also discusses issues of trialability and outlines the benefits of being able to test out new ideas on a small scale before more wide-scale adoption and implementation. This is another issue that is useful for the facilitator to think about: Are there ways in which the evidence or proposed service improvement could be piloted to begin with, for example, through the application of improvement-based Plan–Do–Study–Act (PDSA) cycles?

Recapping what we have discussed so far in relation to the innovation, there appear to be some general considerations related to clarifying the nature of the problem to be addressed, establishing the underlying evidence base and determining how well it fits into the local context, including the stakeholders that are likely to be affected. Box 4.2 summarises the questions that are useful for the facilitator to consider when assessing the characteristics of the innovation.

BOX 4.2   FACILITATION CHECKLIST TO ASSESS THE CHARACTERISTICS OF THE INNOVATION

- Who is likely to be affected by the proposed innovation?
- What is the underlying evidence for the proposed innovation or change?

  - Is it derived from research, clinical consensus, patient views, local information/data – or a combination of these?
  - Is it viewed as rigorous and robust?
  - Is there a shared view about the evidence?
  - How well does it 'fit' the local setting?
  - Is it likely to be accepted or contested by those people who have to implement it?

- Is the evidence packaged in an accessible and usable form, such as a clinical guideline, care pathway or algorithm?

  - Will people be able to see easily and clearly what is proposed in terms of clinical practice and the process of patient care?

- How much novelty does the evidence introduce?

  - Will it require significant changes in the processes and/or systems of care delivery?
  - Will it present a challenge to people's ways of thinking, mental models and relationships?
  - What are the implications of this in terms of the likely boundaries that will be encountered?
  - Will a knowledge transfer, translation or transformation strategy be required?

- Does it offer advantages over the current way of doing things, for example:

  - Will it enhance patient experience?
  - Could it introduce greater efficiency in the provision of care?
  - Will it help to remove bottlenecks in the care process?

- Is there potential to test out/pilot the introduction of the evidence/innovation on a small scale in the first instance?

In order to begin to make sense of the innovation and the changes required to implement it, the facilitator will need to work closely with the recipients of the innovation. As illustrated in Figure 4.3, typical facilitator activities at the level of the innovation will include:

- mapping the stakeholders that will be affected by implementation;
- working with local teams to assess current practice, map processes of care and clarify problems;
- gathering, appraising and synthesising available evidence to inform implementation;
- conducting a preliminary assessment of the local context – including different stakeholder groups – to assess the potential boundaries to knowledge flow and determine likely barriers and enablers of change.

The recipients

As the facilitator starts thinking about the characteristics of the innovation, it is apparent that they begin to move into other levels of the facilitation model; in particular, they have to start thinking about the recipients of the innovation and how they will respond to the changes required to implement the innovation. When we use the term 'recipients', we are referring to the staff, services and patients that will be directly involved in and affected by the implementation process. Having undertaken a baseline assessment, the facilitator should have a general sense of how well the proposed innovation or change is likely to fit into the local setting. Now it is useful to explore issues relating to the recipients in some more depth, particularly in relation to:

- their motivation and ability to change;
- values and beliefs;
- the degree of consensus around the proposed innovation;
- views of local opinion leaders;

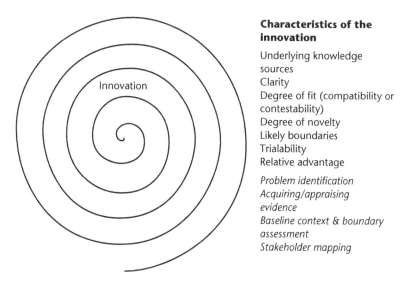

Characteristics of the innovation

Underlying knowledge sources
Clarity
Degree of fit (compatibility or contestability)
Degree of novelty
Likely boundaries
Trialability
Relative advantage

Problem identification
Acquiring/appraising evidence
Baseline context & boundary assessment
Stakeholder mapping

FIGURE 4.3 Facilitation assessment and activity at the level of the innovation

- existing data to inform the change process;
- skills and knowledge;
- time and resources;
- collaboration and teamwork;
- professional boundaries and networks;
- power and authority.

Broadly speaking, these factors can be grouped into thinking about whether the recipients want to implement the innovation (in terms of their motivation, how the innovation fits with their existing practice, values and beliefs, the views of their peers and so on) and whether they can implement the innovation (in that they have the necessary time, resources, knowledge, skills and support). These two elements of 'want to' and 'can do' are drawn from Weiner's theory of organisational readiness to change that we discussed in Chapter 3 (Weiner, 2009). This suggests that organisational readiness depends upon collective behaviour change linked to two key factors, described as change commitment (the 'want to') and change efficacy (the 'can do').

It is also useful to think about what communities of practice exist within the local or clinical setting and how these could affect the proposed innovation in either a supportive or restrictive way. This includes examining the boundaries that exist between different practice communities and what the implications might be from an implementation perspective. Carlile's description of boundaries and how they influence the flow of new knowledge is useful to consider here (Carlile, 2004). For example, is it a relatively simple (syntactic) boundary that needs a shared language to be established (for example, by simplifying some of the clinical terminology), or is it a more complicated boundary which will either require work to find a shared meaning (a semantic boundary), or negotiation and agreement on the changes required to apply the innovation in practice (a pragmatic boundary).

Box 4.3 summarises the reflective questions that the facilitator can use to assess these elements of 'want to' and 'can do' amongst the recipients of the innovation. As you will notice, we are suggesting that these questions should be asked at the level of individual recipients and at the collective level of the team. This is because the theories we considered in Chapter 3 highlighted the importance and influence of peer communication, for example, through working within communities of practice (Wenger, 1998).

BOX 4.3   FACILITATION CHECKLIST TO ASSESS THE RECIPIENT LEVEL OF IMPLEMENTATION

Motivation to change: Individual level

- Do individual members of the team want to apply the change in practice?
- Do they perceive the proposed change as valuable and worthwhile?
- Do they see a need to make the change?
- Is the change consistent with their existing values and beliefs?
- Are there individuals who function as local opinion leaders? Will they be supportive or obstructive in terms of introducing the proposed change?

Motivation to change: Team level

- At a collective level, does the team want to apply the change in practice?
- Is the proposed change seen as valuable and worthwhile?
- Do they see a need to make a change?
- Is there a shared view or are there differences of opinion (e.g. between key individuals or between different professional groups and communities of practice)?
- Is there existing data that can be used to highlight the potential for improvement? Or can you collect data for this purpose?

Ability to change: Individual level

- Are individual members able to implement the proposed change?
- Do they understand what the change entails?
- Is it within their current level of knowledge and skills?
- Will additional training and development be needed?
- Do people understand the modifications that will be needed to routine practice and how to change and embed these?
- Do individuals have the necessary authority to carry out the proposed changes?
- Have key individuals whose support is needed been identified? Are they engaged in discussing and planning implementation?

Ability to change: Team level

- Are the team able to implement the proposed change?
- Do they understand what the change entails?
- Is it within their current level of knowledge and skills?
- Will additional training and development be needed?
- Does the team understand the modifications that will be needed to routine practice and how to change and embed these?
- Does the team have the necessary authority to carry out the proposed changes?
- Is there good interprofessional collaboration and teamwork – between professional groups and between clinical staff and managers?
- Will support be needed to develop more effective collaboration and teamwork?
- Are the potential barriers to implementation known? Are there strategies in place to address these?
- Are the resources available to support the implementation process (e.g. time and/ or financial support for new skills development, new equipment, expert support and advice)?

As well as undertaking this assessment, it is useful to think about what actions the facilitator can take, working with the recipients, to enhance their motivation and ability to implement the innovation. Examples of typical facilitator interventions at the recipient level include the following (Figure 4.4):

- Agreeing the goals of implementation.
- Undertaking a baseline audit to establish the gap between current and desired practice (as defined in the goals).

- Using consensus techniques to review and build a level of agreement for the proposed change.
- Establishing measures that can be used to monitor and evaluate progress with implementation.
- Using improvement methods such as Plan–Do–Study–Act cycles to introduce and test the innovation in practice on a small-scale incremental basis.
- Applying general project and change management principles and methods to plan, structure and resource the implementation process.
- Identifying communities of practice and assessing boundaries.
- Adopting a boundary-spanning role to negotiate boundaries and build links across different professional or stakeholder groups involved in implementation.
- Paying attention to team-building activities to improve collaboration, including addressing issues of conflict management and resolution where necessary.
- Undertaking data collection to develop a deeper understanding of the likely barriers to implementation.

In our own facilitation work, we typically start with the more concrete activities at the innovation–recipient level to establish clarity around the purpose and aims of implementation and the agreed strategies for implementation and evaluation. This is in line with much of the literature on improvement science in healthcare. For example, the Model for Improvement (Langley et al., 1996), which is commonly applied in healthcare improvement, identifies three overarching requirements when planning improvement, namely determining: What are we trying to accomplish (the goals)? How will we know that a change is an improvement (establishing measures and a method of monitoring progress)? What changes can we make that

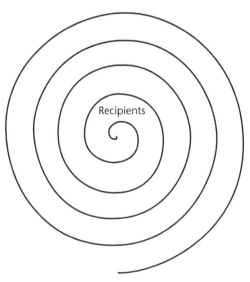

Recipients

Motivation
Values & beliefs
Clinical consensus
Local opinion leaders
Existing data sources
Skills & knowledge
Time & resources
Learning environment
Collaboration & teamwork
Power & authority
Professional boundaries & networks

Goal setting
Consensus building
Audit & feedback
Improvement methods
Project management
Change management
Team building
Conflict management & resolution
Barriers/boundary assessment

FIGURE 4.4 Facilitation assessment and activity at the level of the recipients

will result in improvement (tests of change using PDSA)? Introducing activities such as audit and feedback, process mapping and goal setting at the early stages of implementation helps to enhance the sense of wanting to change amongst the recipients by highlighting the discrepancy between current and desired levels of performance, so creating a sense of dissatisfaction with the status quo and generating a vision for the future.

In parallel to developing a commitment to change, the facilitator also needs to think about the 'can do' issues; in other words, whether those people targeted with the change have confidence in their ability to make the required changes. The level of implementation capability relates to the demands of the task (how complex it is) and the availability of resources (financial, time, skills) to undertake the task. A further important consideration is the process- and team-related issues that are likely to impact upon implementation. This includes thinking about how to use group processes to create a sense of engagement, build consensus and promote more effective collaboration and teamwork. Similarly, where the facilitator identifies sources of resistance or conflict amongst different team members, strategies are needed to address and manage the difficulties or differences of opinion. This may involve the facilitator collecting more detailed information to explore the views of different team members or different stakeholder groups and actively trying to address barriers and span the boundaries between them. In a situation such as this, drawing on something like the Theoretical Domains Framework (TDF) that we described in Chapter 3 is useful to inform a focus group discussion or a series of interviews with key stakeholders (Cane et al., 2012). This provides a set of questions to tap into the 'want to' and 'can do' aspects of implementation, as well as touching on some context-related issues.

One final comment in relation to the recipients of the innovation; as a general aide-memoire, a useful framework for the facilitator is John Adair's model of action-centred leadership (Adair, 1973). Although originally developed as a functional model for group leaders, it provides a simple but helpful guide for facilitators when thinking about implementing the innovation at a recipient level. Basically it suggests that there are three types of needs to be held in balance to achieve the best results. These are described as task, group and individual needs (Figure 4.5). *Task needs* refer to the achievement of agreed goals that are seen as essential for effective group working and are the things that often bring the group together in the first place. *Group needs* are concerned with the way in which the group collectively works together to achieve its goals. *Individual needs* relate to maintaining the motivation and engagement of individual members of the group.

Specific actions that help to address task, group and individual needs are summarised in Table 4.1. However, the key point to emphasise is the need to maintain a balance between the three types of needs. Failure to address one group of needs will eventually impact upon the overall functioning and success of the group. So, for example, imagine that one person totally dominates the group and the facilitator fails to manage that. The problems at the individual level lead to group frustration – maybe some members withdraw from the discussion or stop coming to the meetings – and this eventually reduces the group's effectiveness in meeting its goals. Alternatively, the group may invest a significant time and energy in team-building activities; everyone feels a valued member of the group, but they lose sight of the task. Some people start to question the point of going to meetings as they cannot see any progress being made, which in turn starts to affect the cohesiveness and functioning of the group. What these examples illustrate is that task, group and individual needs are interdependent and lack of attention to one will ultimately have an effect on the others.

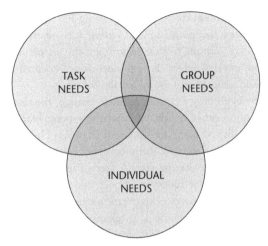

FIGURE 4.5 The inter-relationship between task, group and individual needs After Adair (1973)

TABLE 4.1 Actions to address task, group and individual needs

Task-related action	Group-related action	Individual-related action
• Define the task • Devise a workable plan • Brief team members on the task and their role • Delegate work to team members • Allocate resources • Control the pace of work • Keep the team focused on the plan • Evaluate progress and modify the plan accordingly	• Set ground rules • Lead by example • Build team spirit • Maintain morale • Give encouragement • Motivate members to achieve success • Keep open communication • Deal constructively to resolve conflicts • Avoid getting too deeply embroiled with the task itself	• Involve all team members in discussions and activity • Seek out and use individuals' abilities • Bring in the quieter members • Control overactive members • Establish previous experience • Offer constructive feedback • Praise, support and encourage • Avoid taking sides in an argument

Source: After Adair (1973).

As this table highlights, the facilitator has to juggle a number of different things while working with individuals and teams at a local level to implement an innovation. Knowing how to keep 'all the balls in the air' and when and how to intervene in an appropriate way depends upon making accurate diagnoses of what is happening at a particular point in time and responding accordingly; in turn, this is part of developing the repertoire of facilitation knowledge, skills and experience. A further dimension to the facilitation process is developing an understanding of contextual factors and how best to handle these, both within and outside of the organisation, in terms of their impact upon the implementation of the innovation. We will now turn our attention to these contextual factors, starting with the inner context at the immediate recipient level and the wider organisational level, before looking at factors in the outer health system context.

The inner context: local level

The inner context is concerned with the immediate work environment of the recipients; the ward, practice, unit or department where the innovation is to be implemented. In an organisation-wide implementation project, there may be multiple units or departments involved; however, each will have its own local context and it is important to understand how that influences the processes and outcomes of implementation. In the i-PARIHS framework, we have identified some of the key issues to be considered within the immediate local context, including: formal and informal leadership support, culture, past experience of innovation and change, learning, evaluation and feedback processes and mechanisms for embedding change. A supportive culture for implementing innovation is seen to be one where a humanistic approach to leadership and management is adopted, such that staff and patients feel valued, staff are active participants in decision-making, innovation is encouraged and there is continuous reflection, learning and evaluation, with the necessary supporting structures and processes in place to embed changes in practice. Formal leaders play an important part in creating this type of culture through working in a facilitative and democratic way. Informal leaders may also exist at a professional group or team level and can play an important role in either promoting or potentially blocking proposed innovations in care. Box 4.4 summarises the reflective questions the facilitator can use to assess characteristics of the inner context at a local level.

BOX 4.4   FACILITATION CHECKLIST TO ASSESS THE INNER CONTEXT AT A LOCAL LEVEL

- Who are the formal and informal leaders at a local level?

  - Are they likely to be supportive of the proposed change?
  - Are they helping to create a facilitative context through providing motivation and support, creating a vision and reinforcing the change process?
  - Is there a distributed and devolved style of management?

- Is there a culture that supports innovation and change?

  - Do staff feel actively involved in decisions that affect them?
  - Are staff trusted to introduce new ideas into practice?
  - Do staff and patients feel valued?

- What is the past experience of introducing changes at a local level?
- Is there evidence of ongoing learning and evaluation at a local level?
- Are there mechanisms in place to support learning and evaluation and to embed changes in routine practice (e.g. regular team meetings, audit and feedback processes, professional development opportunities and performance review systems)?

In order to assess the local context, the facilitator has a number of options. They may choose to undertake some observation of the practice environment and interview some of the staff about what it is like to work there. Alternatively, they may opt to survey staff members using a questionnaire approach; or they may decide to use a combination of approaches. A number of instruments based upon the PARIHS framework have been developed and tested to assess contextual factors influencing implementation at a local level. These are summarised in Table 4.2.

TABLE 4.2 Examples of context assessment instruments

Instrument	Brief description
Context Assessment Index (CAI) (McCormack et al., 2009)	37-item instrument that assesses context in relation to five dimensions described as: collaborative practice; evidence-informed practice; respect for persons; practice boundaries; evaluation
Alberta Context Tool (ACT) (Estabrooks et al., 2009)	56–58-item instrument, assessing 10 dimensions of organisational context: leadership; culture; evaluation (feedback processes); social capital; informal interactions; formal interactions; structural and electronic resources; organisational slack – staff; organisational slack – space; organisational slack – time Different versions of the instrument have been developed for different care settings and caregivers
Organisational Change Readiness Assessment (ORCA) (Helfrich et al., 2009)	19-item instrument designed to assess the three core elements of PARIHS: evidence, context and facilitation

Undertaking this more detailed assessment of the local context is one of the practical activities that the facilitator may engage in with the recipients of the innovation. Other facilitator interventions at this level include the following (Figure 4.6):

- Establishing communication and feedback processes to share information about the project to patients, staff and managers at a local level.
- Encouraging networking between the different groups involved in implementation.
- Assessing and spanning the boundaries between patients, professionals and managers.
- Negotiating for resources to support the implementation of the innovation.
- Identifying ways to embed the innovation in local practice.
- Promoting continuous learning and evaluation of the implementation process.

Practical activities to share information about the innovation and its implementation might include producing a poster to display in a prominent area for staff and patients, developing regular project briefings to circulate by email or in printed form, displaying audit results in a simple graphical form to show improvements over time and holding short meetings and presentations to provide updates on implementation to key stakeholder groups. The facilitator and the teams they are working with may also attend existing meetings within the local setting to feedback on the implementation project; in turn, this could help to encourage information sharing and networking between the different stakeholder groups. At a project management level, the facilitator may need to think about calculating what resources are needed to support implementation – in terms of staff, time, skills development, new equipment and so on – and set up meetings with managers and clinical leaders to negotiate for these. Additionally, attention needs to be paid to thinking about how the innovation can be embedded into practice in the longer term to ensure that if and when the facilitation support is withdrawn that practice does not revert to a pre-implementation state. This involves looking at structures and processes

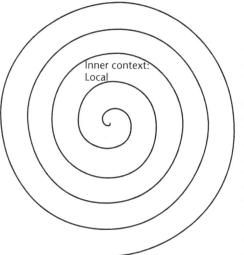

Inner context: local level

Formal & informal leadership support
Culture
Past experience of change
Mechanisms for embedding change
Learning, evaluation & feedback processes
Local context assessment
Communication & feedback
Networking
Boundary assessment & spanning Negotiating & influencing
Policies & procedures
Structuring learning

FIGURE 4.6 Facilitation assessment and activity at the level of the inner–local context

that help integrate the innovation into routine practice, for example, through establishing a regular audit and review process and incorporating new care processes and pathways into local level policies and procedures.

The inner context: organisational level

At the next level of context, we are interested in what factors within the organisational setting might influence the implementation process. These may seem somewhat removed from the specific implementation project with discrete aims, goals and measures; however, there is good evidence to indicate that these types of contextual factors can exert an influence on the processes and outcomes of implementation. At an organisational level, an initial consideration is the extent to which the implementation project is aligned with organisational priorities; where this is the case, there is likely to be greater organisational support for the project, particularly in terms of agreeing the required resources (time, people, finance) to support implementation. The way in which the organisation is structured and managed will impact on how much autonomy local teams have to make decisions about changing systems and processes of care. In a more hierarchically managed organisation, individuals and teams may have less ability to introduce new ideas without going through some kind of formal approval process, which can act to make the implementation process slower and more complex. How the organisation has managed and responded to change in the past is a good indicator of the general culture and receptiveness to innovation and new ideas. Box 4.5 lists the types of questions that the facilitator might want to think about in assessing the organisational context and the likely influence this could have on implementing the innovation.

BOX 4.5 FACILITATION CHECKLIST TO ASSESS THE INNER CONTEXT AT AN ORGANISATIONAL LEVEL

- Do the evidence/innovation and the changes proposed align with the strategic priorities for the organisation?
- Has the support of key individuals and leaders within the organisation been sought and secured?
- Is there a culture that supports innovation and change?
- Is there a history of successful and sustained change within the organisation?
- Does the organisation have systems and processes in place that support innovation and change (e.g. effective information and communication systems, opportunities for networking and learning across departments/teams)?
- Do the senior management team actively seek opportunities for improvement and encourage ideas and feedback from patients, the public and staff?
- Are there mechanisms in place for embedding changes in routine practice (e.g. formal policies and procedures)?

The organisational theories of learning and knowledge management that we considered in Chapter 3 are useful to inform some of this thinking about the organisational context and how it may support or hinder implementation efforts. Generally speaking, organisations that pay more attention to how they use knowledge to inform ongoing reflection and learning are likely to have greater absorptive capacity and provide a more receptive and supportive environment for implementation. From the facilitator's perspective, it is useful to look at how pro-actively the organisation seeks out and uses new knowledge, for example, through participating in learning networks with other organisations, regularly monitoring and evaluating performance at a team and organisational level and analysing and interpreting available data.

Important activities the facilitator can engage in to understand and influence the organisational context level include developing an active communication plan to engage with senior leaders and managers and provide regular feedback on progress (Figure 4.7). It is at this level that the facilitator is likely to take on a more active knowledge-brokering and boundary-spanning role – thinking about the different groups that need to be on board with the project, securing senior level support and sponsorship, targeting key people whose commitment is important and tailoring messages in a way that is appropriate and relevant to the target audience. The facilitator might not be able to directly change the organisational context in which the project is taking place, but they can influence it by the strategic use of communication, networking and negotiation skills. This is particularly important if organisational barriers to implementation are identified.

The outer context

At a wider level still, the facilitator also needs to be aware of the health system in which implementation is taking place, from a political, economic and cultural perspective. Factors such as the presence of policy-drivers that reinforce (or not) the proposed change, regulatory requirements, financial incentives or disincentives to change, the relative stability of the environment and the existence of inter-organisational networks to promote and spread learning are all useful things to take into account (Box 4.6).

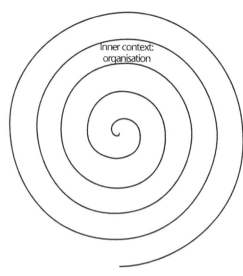

Inner context: local level

Organisational priorities
Structure
Leadership & senior
management support
Systems & processes
Culture
History of innovation & change
Absorptive capacity
Stakeholder engagement
Communication & feedback
Marketing & presentation
Networking
Boundary spanning
Negotiating & influencing
Policies & procedures

FIGURE 4.7 Facilitation assessment and activity at the level of the inner–organisational context

---

BOX 4.6   FACILITATION CHECKLIST TO ASSESS THE OUTER CONTEXT

- Do the evidence/innovation and the changes proposed align with the strategic priorities for the wider health system (e.g. in terms of current health policy, national priorities for action and improvement)?
- Are there incentives in the wider health system that reinforce the proposed change (e.g. pay for performance schemes, regulatory requirements, etc.)?
- Are there inter-organisational networks (e.g. specialised clinical networks) that will be helpful in terms of supporting the proposed changes?
- How much stability/instability is there in the wider health system?
- Is this likely to influence the implementation project?

At this level, the facilitator is even less likely to be able to significantly alter characteristics of the health system, but being aware of what factors are present and how they could act to enable or inhibit the proposed implementation process is crucial. Bate (2014, p.10, citing Waterman, 1987) describes this as a tactic of 'informed opportunism' with regards to the outer context, such as looking to link with a strategy that will help take the innovation forward in the same direction that you want to travel. Take, for example, the case of 'pay for performance' systems. If the implementation project is aligned to one of these schemes, the facilitator could use the financial incentives within the system as a lever for securing engagement and change at a local level. Or, if through the regulatory system the external inspection process traces the uptake of clinical guidelines, the implementation project can be framed as one way of meeting regulatory requirements. The exact nature of the relationship between system level factors and local implementation projects will be determined on a case-by-case basis; the important point is that facilitators need to look at this bigger picture and be politically aware of the health system in which they are operating. Again, this involves engaging in strategic communication and influencing activities, networking across multiple boundaries and developing alliances with key individuals and organisations (Figure 4.8). These activities play an important role in planning for sustainability and spread of the implementation project – something that we will return to and discuss in more detail in Chapter 7.

Putting everything together to create an integrated model of facilitation

As the preceding description illustrates – and Figure 4.2 summarises – when the facilitation role and process is considered in its totality, it is complex, wide-ranging and potentially quite daunting! This raises important questions about who can and should take on the facilitator role, what preparation, development and support they need and how the role should be structured to ensure that it is doable in practice. These are questions we will consider in some more detail as we move through the remaining chapters of the book. As noted at the start of the chapter, remember also that it should not be just one person who has to fulfil all of the different activities that we have outlined at the various levels of implementation. Part of the skill of facilitation is building a team of people who are committed to the same goals and who can share the workload in terms of progressing implementation. The cases we present in subsequent chapters will help to illustrate how this has been achieved in a number of projects in different international and organisational settings.

Summary

In this chapter, we have illustrated a model of facilitation that connects our own experiences with the wider literature on innovation, implementation and change management. The result

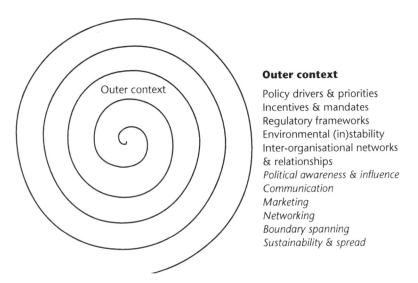

Outer context

Policy drivers & priorities
Incentives & mandates
Regulatory frameworks
Environmental (in)stability
Inter-organisational networks
& relationships
Political awareness & influence
Communication
Marketing
Networking
Boundary spanning
Sustainability & spread

FIGURE 4.8 Facilitation assessment and activity at the level of the outer context

is a goal-centred model of facilitation that is situated in and interacts with the multiple levels that influence – and are influenced by – the process of implementation. A complete checklist of the reflective questions that are useful to consider when planning an implementation project is contained in Appendix 4.1. In the following chapters, we develop the model of facilitation further by focusing more specifically on different facilitator roles from novice through to experienced and expert facilitators. This includes looking at what sort of people make good facilitators, how they get started in the role and what preparation and support is needed on the development journey of a practising facilitator.

References

Adair, J. 1973. *Action-Centred Leadership*. London: McGraw-Hill.

Bate, P. 2014. Context is everything. In: *Perspectives on Context: A Selection of Essays Considering the Role of Context in Successful Quality Improvement*. London: The Health Foundation.

Cane, J., O'Connor, D. & Michie, S. 2012. Validation of the theoretical domains framework for use in behaviour change and implementation research. *Implementation Science*, 7, 37.

Carlile, P.R. 2004. Transferring, translating, and transforming: an integrative framework for managing knowledge across boundaries. *Organization Science*, 15, 555–68.

Dopson, S. & Fitzgerald, L. 2005. *Knowledge to Action? Evidence-Based Health Care in Action*. New York: Oxford University Press.

Estabrooks, C., Squires, J., Cummings, G., Birdsell, J. & Norton, P. 2009. Development and assessment of the Alberta Context Tool. *BMC Health Services Research*, 9, 234.

Ferlie, E., Fitzgerald, L. & Wood, M. 2000. Getting evidence into clinical practice: an organisational behaviour perspective. *Journal of Health Services Research & Policy*, 5, 96–102.

Greenhalgh, T., Robert, G., Macfarlane, F., Bate, P. & Kyriakidou, O. 2004. Diffusion of innovations in service organizations: systematic review and recommendations. *Milbank Quarterly*, 82, 581–629.

Helfrich, C., Li, Y., Sharp, N. & Sales, A. 2009. Organizational readiness to change assessment (ORCA): development of an instrument based on the Promoting Action on Research in Health Services (PARIHS) framework. *Implementation Science*, 4, 38.

Langley, G.J., Nolan, K.M., Norman, C.L., Provost, L.P. & Nolan, T.W. 1996. *The Improvement Guide. A Practical Guide to Enhancing Organisational Performance*. San Francisco: Jossey-Bass.

McCormack, B., McCarthy, G., Wright, J. & Coffey, A. 2009. Development and Testing of the Context Assessment Index (CAI). *Worldviews on Evidence-Based Nursing*, 6, 27–35.

Rogers, E.M. 1995. *Diffusion of Innovations*. New York: The Free Press.

Weiner, B. 2009. A theory of organizational readiness for change. *Implementation Science*, 4, 67.

Wenger, E. 1998. *Communities of Practice: Learning, Meaning and Identity*. Cambridge, UK: Cambridge University Press.

Appendix 4.1 Planning for implementation: A facilitation checklist

When preparing for an implementation project, there are a number of factors that are important to assess – factors that relate to the innovation or change that you are trying to introduce; factors linked to the individuals and teams that you want to adopt the change; and factors concerned with the environment, both internally and externally to the organisation in which implementation is taking place. Use the set of reflective questions below to help you assess and diagnose where you might need to focus attention in terms of facilitating the implementation process.

1. Characteristics of the innovation

- Who is likely to be affected by the proposed innovation?
- What is the underlying evidence for the proposed innovation or change?

  o Is it derived from research, clinical consensus, patient views, local information/data – or a combination of these?
  o Is it viewed as rigorous and robust?
  o Is there a shared view about the evidence?
  o How well does it 'fit' the local setting?
  o Is it likely to be accepted or contested by those people who have to implement it?

- Is the evidence packaged in an accessible and usable form (e.g. a clinical guideline, care pathway or algorithm)?

  o Will people be able to see easily and clearly what is proposed in terms of clinical practice and the process of patient care?

- How much novelty does the evidence introduce?

  o Will it require significant changes in the processes and/or systems of care delivery?
  o Will it present a challenge to people's ways of thinking, mental models and relationships?
  o What are the implications of this in terms of the likely boundaries that will be encountered?
  o Will a knowledge transfer, translation or transformation strategy be required?

- Does it offer advantages over the current way of doing things, for example:

  o Will it enhance patient experience?
  o Could it introduce greater efficiency in the provision of care?
  o Will it help to remove bottlenecks in the care process?

- Is there potential to test out/pilot the introduction of the evidence/innovation on a small scale in the first instance?

2. The recipients of the evidence/innovation

Think about the people who you want to implement the change and how they are likely to respond – both at an individual level and as a member of a clinical or service delivery team. Reflect on whether they want to introduce the innovation and if they are able to implement the required changes.

2a. Motivation to change: Individual level

- Do individual members of the team want to apply the change in practice?
- Do they perceive the proposed change as valuable and worthwhile?
- Do they see a need to make the change?
- Is the change consistent with their existing values and beliefs?
- Are there individuals who function as local opinion leaders? Will they be supportive or obstructive in terms of introducing the proposed change?

2b. Motivation to change: Team level

- At a collective level, does the team want to apply the change in practice?
- Is the proposed change seen as valuable and worthwhile?
- Do they see a need to make a change?
- Is there a shared view or are there differences of opinion (e.g. between key individuals or between different professional groups and communities of practice)?
- Is there existing data that can be used to highlight the potential for improvement? Or can you collect data for this purpose?

2c. Ability to change: Individual level

- Are individual members able to implement the proposed change?

  o Do they understand what the change entails?
  o Is it within their current level of knowledge and skills?
  o Will additional training and development be needed?

- Do people understand the modifications that will be needed to routine practice and how to change and embed these?
- Do individuals have the necessary authority to carry out the proposed changes?
- Have key individuals whose support is needed been identified? Are they engaged in discussing and planning implementation?

2d. Ability to change: Team level

- Are the team able to implement the proposed change?

  o Do they understand what the change entails?
  o Is it within their current level of knowledge and skills?
  o Will additional training and development be needed?

- Does the team understand the modifications that will be needed to routine practice and how to change and embed these?
- Does the team have the necessary authority to carry out the proposed changes?
- Is there good inter-professional collaboration and teamwork – between professional groups and between clinical staff and managers?
- Will support be needed to develop more effective collaboration and teamwork?
- Are the potential barriers to implementation known? Are there strategies in place to address these?

- Are the resources available to support the implementation process, for example: time and/or financial support for new skills development, new equipment, expert support and advice?

3. The inner context

Think about the characteristics of the context in which the innovation is to be implemented – both the immediate local context in which the recipients are working and the wider organisational context in which their unit or department operates.

3a. The local context

- Who are the formal and informal leaders at a local level?

   o   Are they likely to be supportive of the proposed change?
   o   Are they helping to create a facilitative context through providing motivation and support, creating a vision and reinforcing the change process?
   o   Is there a distributed and devolved style of management?

- Is there a culture that supports innovation and change?

   o   Do staff feel actively involved in decisions that affect them?
   o   Are staff trusted to introduce new ideas into practice?
   o   Do staff and patients feel valued?

- What is the past experience of introducing changes at a local level?
- Are there mechanisms in place to support learning and evaluation and to embed changes in routine practice (e.g. regular team meetings, audit and feedback processes, professional development opportunities and performance review systems)?

3b. The organisational context

- Do the evidence/innovation and the changes proposed align with the strategic priorities for the organisation?
- Has the support of key individuals and leaders within the organisation been sought and secured?
- Is there a culture that supports innovation and change?
- Is there a history of successful and sustained change within the organisation?
- Does the organisation have systems and processes in place that support innovation and change (e.g. effective information and communication systems, opportunities for networking and learning across departments/teams)?
- Do the senior management team actively seek opportunities for improvement and encourage ideas and feedback from patients, the public and staff?
- Are there mechanisms in place for embedding changes in routine practice (e.g. formal policies and procedures)?

4. The outer context

Consider what is happening in the wider health system that might affect the inner context. Although it may not be possible to directly influence the outer context, it is important to be aware of how the outer context might impact upon local implementation – and whether this creates opportunities from which the project might be able to gain leverage.

- Do the evidence/innovation and the changes proposed align with the strategic priorities for the wider health system (e.g. in terms of current health policy, national priorities for action and improvement)?
- Are there incentives in the wider health system that reinforce the proposed change (e.g. pay for performance schemes, regulatory requirements, etc.)?
- Are there inter-organisational networks (e.g. specialised clinical networks) that will be helpful in terms of supporting the proposed changes?
- How much stability/instability is there in the wider health system?

    o   Is this likely to influence the implementation project?

5

GETTING STARTED WITH FACILITATION

The facilitator's role

Alison Kitson and Gill Harvey

Introduction

In the previous chapters we have outlined the development and use of the PARIHS framework. We have also outlined our revised PARIHS framework that we are calling the integrated or i-PARIHS framework.

Our refined PARIHS framework has kept the centrality of facilitation. The 'i' in i-PARIHS stands for integration of these new ingredients (innovation, recipients and inner and outer context) through skilled facilitation. Facilitation is the active ingredient in the original PARIHS framework and it has remained the active ingredient in the i-PARIHS framework. Facilitation is a deliberate and conscious process that can be taught and refined through practice and reflection. It can be a unique role or it can be a set of skills and attributes that a person incorporates into an existing role such as a clinical leader or an educator.

In this chapter we will focus on what facilitation is and what sort of people become facilitators. We will then look at how facilitators differ from other knowledge translation, implementation or change management roles. The chapter concludes by providing a pathway from novice facilitator to experienced and expert facilitator. We will illustrate each of the sections in the chapter with findings from studies we have been involved in over the years.

By the end of the chapter the reader should be in a better position to understand why facilitation is the central part of the process of successfully getting new ideas into everyday practice. In addition, the reader should be able to identify what skills they have that could enable them to take a more facilitative approach to their work and also to think more systematically about developing new skills and attributes when they are introducing evidence into practice.

What is facilitation?

In previous chapters we have described how our experiences around helping clinicians and others introduce new ideas and evidence into practice led us to conclude that the processes involved were more about enabling, negotiating and supporting change rather than telling people what to do. In Chapter 4 we have begun to outline the ways in which the i-PARIHS framework can be operationalised through the process of facilitation. In simple terms, facilitation is defined as a process of enabling groups or teams to work effectively together to achieve a common goal (Schwarz, 2002). Facilitation as a method of supporting change in the way individuals think and act is not unique to the evidence-based healthcare movement or to knowledge translation activities. Indeed, the concept of facilitation can be traced to three different philosophical traditions.

The first of these is humanistic psychology, where facilitation approaches have been used to shape counselling and therapeutic client-centred approaches. Carl Rogers' work has also influenced the crossover of these humanistic principles to inform educational approaches, particularly in adult learning (Rogers, 1969). Peter Reason and John Heron both looked at shaping the learning experience of groups based on these humanistic principles (Reason, 1988; Heron, 1989), as well as principles for educational psychology and action science. Champions of the action science approach to facilitation were people like Donald Schon and Chris Argyris (Schon, 1983; Argyris and Schon, 1996) who led the movement around practice-based learning or learning from experience. For them, facilitation was the mechanism through which individuals and groups could be enabled to learn from practice and, importantly, to co-create new knowledge through critical dialogue between the practitioner (learner) and the facilitator (the expert enabler of learning).

The third main area to influence our thinking around facilitation has been the broad field of organisational psychology and in particular theories relating to how organisations learn and improve what they do. Argyris and Schon demonstrated the importance of recognising and acknowledging the individual in the system and how by unlocking their ability to reflect on their everyday practices they could improve what they did (Argyris and Schon, 1996). Similar principles are embedded in quality improvement theories (Deming, 2000) and theories of innovation and organisational change (Van de Ven et al., 1999; Van de Ven, 2007). For Deming, the ability of the individual to influence change was structured within a process re-engineering framework. The skill of facilitation was to balance the system improvement with the changes that needed to be created within the ways of working and relationships between team members. Van de Ven also identified the importance of collaboration between different groups of experts and termed the phrase 'engaged scholarship' to reflect the importance of the external expert role in enabling and supporting the activities of the team and organisation to be innovative (Van de Ven, 2007).

Facilitation is thus a well-recognised enabling process, which, as we have just described, has its origins in a range of different philosophical backgrounds and theories. Despite the interest in facilitation, it would be accurate to say that there are no clear or definitive descriptions of exactly what it is and how to teach it, particularly as it is used in evidence-based healthcare or knowledge translation activity. What we intend to do in this chapter is to begin to lay out our approach to facilitation, based on our experience and feedback from multiple studies.

Facilitation enables a shared understanding of a task or activity. It involves key players in an active way through enabling meaningful participation and ownership of one's actions. This ability to help individuals feel in control and empowered leads to purposeful and collective action that creates the change or improvement. The emphasis is therefore on relationships, learning, and shared problem-solving. Facilitation within the i-PARIHS framework also uses the structure of looking at the nature of the evidence or innovation, paying attention to the recipients of the innovation being introduced and considering the context, both the local or inner context and the wider or outer context. Box 5.1 summarises the main characteristics of facilitation within the i-PARIHS framework.

BOX 5.1 CHARACTERISTICS OF FACILITATION WITHIN THE i-PARIHS FRAMEWORK

- Participation and involvement of key stakeholders
- Ownership and control of the process by those responsible for change
- Problem-focused and discrete
- System-sensitive
- Integrated and iterative
- Linking local initiatives to wider system changes
- Providing feedback on activity through simple 'real-time' mechanisms
- Empowering and enabling others
- Managing group dynamics

What does a 'good' facilitator look like?

In our work we have been able to collect information from individuals who have chosen to be facilitators or have been asked to facilitate a piece of evidence or an innovation into their work activity. In answering the question of what a good facilitator looks like, we will draw on data from several workshops we have been involved in running where we explored this question. To answer the question we developed a structured process where participants involved in facilitation could reflect on their personal experiences of either doing the facilitation or being facilitated by someone else. As well as exploring the tacit knowledge and experience held by practitioners we wanted to try to create descriptors (or typologies) that would lead to identifying core elements of facilitation. The data were collected from four workshop events run by the lead author between 2008 and 2009. A total of 89 participants responded to the exercise and these respondents came from Ireland (14), Australia (15) and Canada (60).

At the workshops, the goal was to use an interactive, experiential-based facilitative approach to elicit the tacit knowledge of the participants as a way of understanding the skill, knowledge and expertise participants had around facilitation and then to identify ways of developing new skills and approaches. The approach was structured in six steps.

The first step required participants, prior to the facilitation workshop they were attending, to complete a template where they described two experiences: one where they experienced positive facilitation and one where the experience was not positive. No definitions, prompts or direction were given at this time. Then, at the workshop (step 2), before any discussion about facilitation, participants were grouped into teams of three people (or triads). Each participant had the opportunity to share both the positive and negative experiences. The third step was to involve the triads in theming their key phrases to create larger categories for both positive and negative experiences (step 4). The categories were then shared across the whole workshop (step 5), and participants had the opportunity to look for patterns and themes emerging from their collective experiences. The final step (step 6) was where the whole group divided into teams of six participants. The new teams had the task of reading through the collective work (either positive or negative accounts) and creating a 'story' that reflected the 'essence' or essential elements of the characteristics of good and not so good facilitation. The stories became the exemplars or 'archetypes' connecting participants' tacit (intuitive, implicit and emotional) experiences of facilitation with their intellectual, rational understanding of facilitation.

Participants were self-selected in that they had chosen or were part of a hospital- or organisational-wide initiative around getting new evidence into practice in their respective countries. This meant that they should have had some prior experience in facilitation roles. However, this was not a requirement and the workshops were designed to create agreement across the participants around what they thought was important in facilitation. Output from each workshop was synthesised and sent to workshop participants for validation and then the data from all four workshops were collated to provide a summary of the main findings.

A number of consistent themes emerged from the data, which described both positive and negative facilitation experiences. Positive facilitation experiences derived from facilitators who were able to do the following things:

- Clarify the task in hand.
- Be clear who the key stakeholders were and how they needed to be engaged.
- Clarify who needed to be in the team, and how it was going to work.
- Demonstrate the specific skill-set required.
- Know how to engage emotionally as well as intellectually with the proposed change.
- Be able to engage participants as individuals.

These characteristics were part of what it meant to be a 'good' facilitator. Table 5.1 details the other elements thought to be important around each main characteristic.

Negative experiences or poor facilitation, as perhaps expected, were often described as the lack of the above characteristics. These were a lack of clarity around task and stakeholders, lack of ownership and control of the innovation or project, poor team dynamics, lack of trust, lack of knowledge and skills, poor planning or preparation, negative emotions, poor communication and failure to link the specific initiative with wider organisational contextual issues such as politics, resources, priorities, timeliness and overall patient benefit. Table 5.2 summarises these findings.

What we have shown in summarising this piece of work is that facilitation is recognised as a mechanism and is commonly understood within health systems that are actively working on introducing new innovations and evidence into practice. The individuals who choose to or who are selected to become facilitators have themselves experienced positive and negative facilitation processes. These experiences can be used to help improve the overall quality of the facilitation experience and provide more structured support to individuals who become facilitators. The purpose of this book is to begin to systematically describe effective facilitation approaches and to enable facilitators to embark on a more structured learning journey.

What sort of people become facilitators?

We still have to say something about the sorts of people who choose to become facilitators. Again, this role can be an explicit role (as described in earlier chapters where we outlined facilitators as part of quality improvement, leadership or practice development initiatives), or it can be a time-limited project officer role where a clinical staff member, often a nurse, is asked to undertake a particular time-limited project. What we also want to stress is the essential 'attributes' of facilitation as well as the essential 'tasks' that need to be undertaken. Facilitators have both a set of personal characteristics that predispose them to choose the role and they also need to have a set of skills and abilities that will help them master the tasks involved in managing

TABLE 5.1 Characteristics of positive facilitation and good facilitators

Clarity around the task	• Characteristics such as novelty, complexity • Purpose • Relevance • Timeliness • Focus • Culturally sensitive • Clear expectations
Clarity around stakeholders	• Students/patients/nurses/multi-disciplinary team • Presence, availability, engaging, consent • Managers – ensure facilitator has authority
Clarity around team	• Role, knowledge, readiness, group dynamics • Valuing input, inclusion, respect, collaboration • Group readiness
Skill-set of facilitator	• Credible knowledge base for both content and processes • Project management skills • Reflective practitioner • Empowers others • Unbiased • Respectful • Active listener • Builds trust • Able to arrive at decisions and actions • Uses simple materials • Sets ground rules • Good communication skills • Prepares • Know how to appraise the evidence • Emotional engagement – dismisses fears and manages expectations
Communication	• Frequent, consistent messages shared • Clarity • Simplicity • Timeliness
Resources	• Able to do what you have been asked to do • Feedback and evaluation
Leadership and planning	• Timing • Resources • Management support – empowering the facilitator and giving them authority to act
Characteristics of participants	• Active learning • Interpersonal relations • Self-discovery
Personal development	• Equal opportunities • Professional development

TABLE 5.2 Characteristics of inappropriate facilitation and poor facilitators

Lack of clarity around task and stakeholders	• Participants come with different agendas • Different priorities • Unrealistic expectations • Objectives and outcomes not clear
Lack of ownership and control	• No voice • Defensive behaviour not managed • Negative power relationships interfering with the process
Poor team dynamics	• Poor group processes • Group expectations not set or met • Ground rules not established
Lack of trust	• Time not spent in building relations • Participants not able to get to know each other • Feeling isolated and unvalued
Lack of knowledge and skills	• In process • In facilitation
Poor planning and preparation	• Case not made for change • Purpose/goal not clear • Lack of preparation
Negative emotions	• Clashes with values and beliefs • Not knowing how to resolve negative emotions in groups • Managing conflict and anger badly
Poor communication	• Not listening • Technology not working
Wider context	• Politics not acknowledged or managed • Timeliness and appropriateness not considered within wider context • Benefit unclear • Resources lacking

the processes. From the workshops we found clear attributes of facilitation which we termed 'being a facilitator', as opposed to the process of facilitation which was more about 'doing' facilitation. The being and doing dimensions reflect the early differentiation in the original PARIHS framework around attributes (being) and role and purpose (doing). It is important to ensure the right mix or balance of these two key dimensions (Table 5.3).

How do facilitators differ from other helping roles?

We have made the case that the facilitator's role is to make things easier for others through clarifying what has to be done, how best to do it and how to reflect and learn from that process. A facilitator helps individuals, teams or groups of people understand their common objectives and assists them in achieving those objectives without taking responsibility for the action. Facilitators enable more harmonious group work by understanding group dynamics and by optimising the intellectual and problem-solving capabilities of individuals and of the group.

TABLE 5.3 'Being' a facilitator and 'doing' facilitation

NATURE 'being it': Essential 'attributes'	PROCESS 'doing it': Essential 'tasks'
• Realistic • Pragmatic • Fearless • Courageous • Patient • Resilient • Operating with reciprocity • Curious • Promotes discovery • Organic • Comfortable with ambiguity • Able to manage dissonance and conflict	• Identifying and responding to an issue of importance • Knowing how to translate evidence into useful pieces • Expert in managing processes • Knowing how to engage and teach others • Knowing how to build consensus and promote effective teamwork • Diagnosing the issues • Getting things done in a timely manner

The emphasis of the facilitator's role is on helping rather than telling, thus the facilitator supports the process of implementation through the use of a range of structured methods and tools, rather than telling people what they need to change and why. As we will see later there are a number of standard tools and techniques for facilitators, ranging from what the beginner or novice facilitator should know, right through to the advanced skills and knowledge of the expert facilitator.

As we noted earlier, many people implicitly understand the importance of facilitation and have a working knowledge of either being a facilitator or being facilitated. This style of 'getting things done' is consistent with modern leadership approaches, particularly those that promote a learning organisation culture, embrace distributed and transformational leadership behaviours and value and respect the contribution of the workforce. In such organisations, facilitation approaches would be expected in leadership positions and in project management or change initiatives. However, it would be fair to say that this is not the norm in many healthcare organisations, where leadership approaches may tend to be more hierarchical and bureaucratic in nature. If this is the case then the facilitation approach described here will be more alien to the prevailing organisational culture. This would mean that any change or project management approach could be more directive in style. This is not a problem, so long as the facilitator in charge of the implementation process is aware of the constraints and the potential challenge of introducing many of the standard facilitation mechanisms and processes.

The plethora of roles that have developed over the years to aid the implementation of evidence and innovations into health systems reflects this diversity of ideology and approach to change. At one extreme there would be the directive, task-focused, instrumental approach to implementation. These roles could link to individuals whose job it is to enforce mandatory standards, undertake risk audits and reviews and to accredit organisations. At the other extreme would be emancipatory practice development facilitators who would target the individual's personal development as the primary organisational goal. In the middle would be numerous roles that have grown up around the desire to ensure that the new knowledge or evidence is spread across the organisation. These roles are variously described as information and exchange officers, boundary spanners, academic detailers or data linkage personnel. The emphasis here is on the information, not the individual receiving it or the ability of the system to manage the process.

Staff in legitimate leadership roles, as stated earlier, can demonstrate facilitative characteristics as they take responsibility for achieving the change. The formal facilitator's role does not take the responsibility away from the local leaders and their teams to internalise and own the new innovation. This is an important point to make as often, with novice facilitators who may not have a lot of support and are working in an organisation that may not be fully receptive to facilitation principles, the responsibility for delivery is put onto the facilitator rather than the team that the facilitator is enabling.

Table 5.4 summarises some of the main roles in implementation and knowledge translation, including the similarities and differences between facilitators and other enabling and leadership roles.

A growing amount of research has been undertaken on these roles. Different professional groups tend to favour different approaches. Much of the work on opinion leaders has been carried out in medicine, where it was found that the introduction of new evidence can be significantly improved by identifying and using internal opinion leaders (Lomas et al., 1991). It is interesting to note that when this study was replicated in maternity nursing, one of the major challenges was that it was difficult to identify who the local opinion leaders were (Hodnett et al., 1996). This suggests that different professional groups may have different experiences and expectations in terms of how change is implemented and managed.

The Cochrane Effective Practice and Organisation of Care review (EPOC) group has also explored different roles (http://www.epoc.cochrane.org/). Consistent limitations emerge around the difficulty of clearly describing the role being used to support implementation (whether that be a facilitator, knowledge broker, boundary spanner or opinion leader), followed by ensuring the 'fidelity' (or how the role does what it is supposed to do) of the role descriptors when a project or study is being undertaken. What may be a more useful way of thinking about these different roles is not to see them as competing but to recognise their main focus for change. So, for example, opinion leaders and similar roles focus on the recipient of the new knowledge (mostly at the individual level). Intuitively they know how important it is to shape human behaviour by being an example of what the future should look like. In contrast, academic detailers and project managers focus on a particular task in the overall process. This is usually a prescribed role embedded within a way of looking at the new knowledge as a piece of information that has to be imparted in a technical, instrumental way. For the range of roles that pay attention to how new knowledge moves across boundaries (knowledge and exchange workers, boundary spanners, knowledge managers, linkage and exchange workers), the primary focus is on how to optimise the movement of particular pieces of knowledge across systems, groups and teams in order to embed it in individuals and teams.

What is important to make explicit in our focus on facilitation is that we would argue that the good facilitator is drawing on all of these approaches to be able to achieve successful implementation of a new piece of knowledge or innovation into practice. Again, note that the predominant roles reflect the dimensions of the i-PARIHS framework. Characteristics of the innovation are addressed by those roles focused on getting the knowledge right; getting the individuals and systems on board is the remit of the opinion leaders and change champions, while the knowledge and exchange roles focus on inner and outer contextual issues and the way knowledge moves around the system. In our final section of this chapter we will outline how facilitation can embrace all of these dimensions in a systematic way. This is the facilitation journey. Chapters 6 and 7 will describe the steps involved in further detail.

TABLE 5.4 Different roles involved in implementation and knowledge translation

Main role	Description	Alignment to the facilitator role
Opinion leaders	Identified early on in research into the diffusion of innovations, opinion leaders are individuals who possess authority and credibility to shape and influence other colleagues. Through their leadership they can encourage and motivate individuals to change the way they think and behave	Certainly, an important part of being able to shape and influence what individuals think, and how they might be persuaded to change what they do. However, the opinion leader is not explicitly responsible for thinking about how individuals and groups gain knowledge and insight into making the change happen. They are more the catalysts for negotiating that change is needed and open the way for a more structured approach
Academic detailers	This role has emerged from studies in medical sociology looking at how physicians could change their prescribing practices. Academic detailers are trained up to impart specific knowledge to key target groups to change their behaviours and practices. They are not seen as credible internal opinion leaders, more as information providers	The structured learning around the new knowledge/evidence and how to impart it would be consistent with the structured learning approach of the facilitator. The academic detailer role would be external to the organisation and would be formal in terms of the way of engaging with the local individuals and teams. There would be no expectation that the academic detailer role would be considering wider team dynamics or process issues
Knowledge brokers	This role sits between knowledge producers (e.g. scientists and researchers) and people who use the knowledge (e.g. policy-makers, consumers, patients, healthcare professionals). They are used particularly in organisations that are involved in the transfer of technologies to commercialisation	The idea of knowledge brokers moving information from one part of the healthcare system to another has been used in public health in particular. The role of the knowledge brokers is to get the information to the people who need it. There is no expectation that they are required to help the users understand and apply it
Boundary spanners	People who connect different parts of the organisation together to spread innovations and ideas. They monitor and scan the environment as well as transfer technology and information across boundaries	The focus of the boundary spanner's role is to ensure the necessary knowledge moves effectively through the organisation, in particular traversing the many intersections which may or may not be responsive to the new knowledge. They would work across departments and organisations and as such would reflect the stakeholder management and attention to local cultures and contexts that facilitators need to employ

Knowledge managers	People employed, usually in industry, to manage 'knowledge' which is seen as an asset. Their role embraces both the technological and social networking requirements of knowledge management	The knowledge manager's focus is on the movement of appropriate knowledge across the organisation. They generally do not have responsibility for ensuring that recipients use that knowledge resource effectively. A facilitator would use aspects of a knowledge manager's skill-set, particularly around social networks and establishing communities of practice to help embed and sustain innovations
Project managers	Individuals responsible for accomplishing the stated objectives of a project. Part of their role involves setting clear goals, building project requirements, managing constraints and challenges and ensuring quality of the process	A necessary part of the facilitator's skill repertoire is to have good project management skills, particularly around clarity of task, managing deadlines, constraints and challenges. Importantly, the facilitator's role is to enable others to develop these skills
Change champions	People who voluntarily take special interest in the adoption, implementation and use of an issue, programme, idea, policy or project. They help to get the idea accepted at local level. Similar to opinion leaders in many ways	Facilitators would actively recruit change champions to help spread the new idea and embed it. The main point of difference is that facilitators are recruited into the role while change champions are self-selecting volunteers

The facilitator's journey

We need to go back to a couple of terms used in earlier chapters and in particular the ways in which the facilitator role has developed and matured. In the original Standards of Care work (Royal College of Nursing, 1990) we described three different roles: local, key and external facilitators. Local facilitators were individuals recruited to work directly with individuals and teams in their own locality. The other members of the teams knew them and they were sufficiently respected, with the authority to take on the role of local facilitator. Key facilitators were more experienced and senior individuals in the organisation who supported and mentored local facilitators, combining the practical activity on the ground with the more systemic, political activity involved in making change happen at the local level. External facilitators were external to the organisation or health system and were often the expert mentor or consultant supporting and guiding the facilitation effort. External facilitators could be academics, researchers or consultants.

Stetler et al. (2006) subsequently divided the facilitator roles into internal facilitators and external facilitators. In their description internal facilitators would include both local and key facilitators, whereas external covers any facilitator who does not belong to the organisation or health system where the facilitation is happening.

What we are proposing is a journey for the facilitator to go from a novice facilitator to the final destination of becoming an expert facilitator (Figure 5.1). Table 5.5 describes the main characteristics of the role at different points of the journey.

It is possible to start out on the facilitation journey as an external novice facilitator, a stranger to the organisation, team or unit where you will be working. Equally, you may be asked to take on a role of facilitating a change in practice where you are working with your colleagues in your own unit. Here you would be an internal novice facilitator. Being an outsider is sometimes easier than having to facilitate people whom you know. These subtle differences

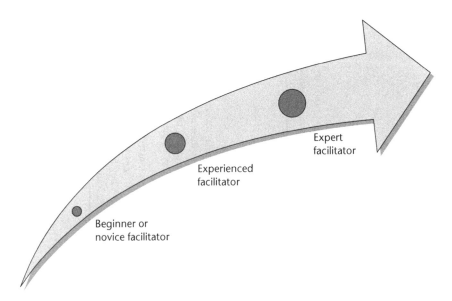

FIGURE 5.1 The facilitator's journey

TABLE 5.5 Novice, experienced and expert facilitators

Experience	Focus of facilitation
Novice facilitator	Working under the supervision of an experienced facilitator and mentored by an expert facilitator Focus on: • What an innovation is; what evidence there is; how to assess evidence • What motivates individuals; how teams work • What context is; what impact context has on implementation at a local level; context at wider organisational level Learning and development around: • Basic skills of facilitation: clarify and engage; assess and measure; action and implementation; review and share • Beginning to build up repertoire of comparing organisational contexts and cultures • Learning how to speed up/refine certain processes • Networking people across sites and building capacity • Embedding innovations into organisational infrastructure • Understanding how to sustain the innovation and promote its spread across the system • Knowing how to measure impact
Experienced facilitator	Working under the supervision of an expert facilitator In-depth understanding and knowledge of the organisation or organisations they are working with Awareness of competing tensions and how to manage these around innovations In-depth understanding of individual motivations and productivity Knowledge of team motivation and productivity Experienced and knowledgeable in local context evaluation Able to assess system-wide activities and influence actions Aware of wider contextual issues and confident in terms of managing boundaries and political tensions Advanced skills of facilitation around the four phases of the Facilitator's Toolkit: clarify and engage; assess and measure; action and implementation; review and share
Expert facilitator	Expert facilitator operating as a guide and mentor to other facilitators Mentoring and coaching experienced facilitators Coordinating facilitation networks Working with systems to improve implementation success Working across academic, service and other organisational boundaries to integrate facilitation and research activity Developing and testing theories of implementation, innovation and facilitation Evaluating interventions Generating new knowledge Refining and improving learning materials and mentoring processes Running workshops and advanced master classes on facilitation approaches

and challenges will be discussed in more detail in the next two chapters as well as in the case study chapters. It is also important to emphasise the need for ongoing mentoring and support for facilitator roles. The development process should ideally move individuals and teams from relative beginners to experts in implementation and evaluation techniques. Unfortunately, the reality is sometimes rather different.

Why making this journey explicit is important: the lone facilitator's story

All too often we hear stories or are involved in programmes to introduce new evidence or knowledge into practice that are less than perfect in their execution. By making the steps more explicit we argue that the success rate for successful implementation will be improved and we will also be able to collect more robust data of effect and understand why things did or did not work well. To illustrate this point, we describe the following case study that involved a novice facilitator who was asked to undertake a hospital-wide implementation programme without a structured support programme around her.

A senior clinical nurse with over 20 years' experience had undertaken a small study within the hospital as part of her personal and professional development and had really enjoyed the challenge. She was subsequently asked to be the project lead for the hourly rounding project and was given six months to ensure that the whole nursing workforce across one large tertiary hospital had implemented the project. Elliott (2014) describes how the individual undertook a reflective journey with two clinical researchers acting as 'critical companions' to help draw out what was happening along the journey, how the individual could manage the size of the task and how they could learn from what worked and what could have been improved. A single descriptive case study framework (Yin, 2009) was used for the research, which was conducted longitudinally across the timeline of the implementation project. A series of interviews were undertaken in which the participant described her experience of being a lone facilitator.

The individual in the study was not an experienced facilitator and although keen to expand her role, she was not given any formal training or support to take the lead on the project. Little formal assessment or planning was undertaken in terms of scoping the size, complexity and resource required to do the work. This became clear to the lone facilitator as she embarked on the preparation and implementation phases. However, from the series of interviews conducted with her, it was clear that she felt personally responsible and at risk if the project was not successful or did not meet its deadlines.

These pressures added to her anxiety and feeling of isolation. Several of the themes to emerge from the study reflect this anxiety – 'being alone', 'self-doubt', 'learning as I go', 'making time and achieving little', 'negative self-description', credibility', 'personal cost'. These were contrasted with more affirmative statements as personal confidence built up during the course of the project, including 'hope and optimism', 'motivation', 'personal commitment', 'personal and professional development' and getting to grips with the size and complexity of the task.

The overriding message from the study was to question the organisational wisdom of initiating significant implementation projects without due consideration of the size, complexity and timeframe, as well as consideration of the support and training required by the project lead. It was also clear (to the research team at least) that the lone facilitator's role was a mix of a project lead and a facilitator and enabler of other staff members' behaviour. The lone facilitator did not have a formal team of local champions or local facilitators to help move the work on across the organisation and the consequence of this seemed to be that she had to operate at all levels within the organisation, undertaking work with local groups as well as coordinating a hospital-wide plan.

Despite the challenges and the obvious stress, the lone facilitator did find the experience a valuable one.

'I mean, now I'm not just a ward nurse; I'm a hospital nurse' (Interview 5)

This is an important statement, as it tends to encapsulate the sort of individuals who choose to take on more formal facilitation roles. They are individuals who reflect the personal qualities of professionalism, commitment to patient care and improvement, are open and generous in enabling others to develop and learn and they are ready to expand their own influence across the organisation or network. Most importantly, from this case study, we can demonstrate the relevance of many of the elements from the earlier study. For example, the need to clarify roles, responsibilities, the scope and nature of the task and to ensure that the facilitator has the requisite skill-set to do the job or – if a novice facilitator – that they are mentored and sup-ported in their activity. Also of note is the fact that facilitation is rarely a lone activity. It should be part of an organisational development process that identifies individuals in the organisation who are ready for a developmental challenge and who can then be supported to do that in a structured and systematic way.

Summary

This chapter has focused on facilitation and the facilitator role. Central to the new i-PARIHS framework, the facilitator role enacts the way that innovations are implemented in order to improve care. Embodied in the facilitator's understanding and actions is the ability to bring groups together and manage a project. The facilitator also has a clear set of personal charac-teristics which promote trust, respect and willingness from others to want to work with them. Facilitation skills need to be developed and refined within a mentoring and support system: novice facilitators are supported by experienced or expert facilitators. Facilitators can either operate in their own organisation (internal facilitators) or they can work in other groups, units or organisations where they do not normally belong (external facilitators). Both internal and external facilitator roles have benefits and challenges. These will be discussed in later chapters.

Most important is the need for facilitators of evidence-based innovation to be supported in their activity. Facilitation is a complex and sophisticated task and it is important to ensure the correct development and support as identified in the studies described in this chapter. We will move on to outline exactly how the novice facilitator can begin their journey of developing the necessary skills and abilities to move from a novice facilitator to an experienced facilitator.

References

Argyris, C. & Schon, D.A. 1996. *Organizational Learning II: Theory, Method and Practice*. Reading, MA: Addison-Wesley.

Deming, W.E. 2000. *Out of the Crisis*. Cambridge, MA: MIT Press.

Elliott, J. 2014. How does an acute care setting respond to a national directive in introducing an organizational wide innovation? A descriptive single case study. Master of Nursing Science, Adelaide, University of Adelaide.

Heron, J. 1989. *The Facilitator's Handbook*. London: Kogan Page.

Hodnett, E.D., Kaufman, K., O'Brien-Pallas, L., Chipman, M., Watson-Macdonell, J. & Hunsburger, W. 1996. A strategy to promote research-based nursing care: effects on childbirth outcomes. *Research in Nursing & Health*, 19, 13–20.

Lomas, J., Enkin, M., Anderson, G.M., Hannah, W.J., Vayda, E. & Singer, J. 1991. Opinion leaders vs audit and feedback to implement practice guidelines: delivery after previous cesarean section. *Journal of the American Medical Association*, 265, 2202–207.

Reason, P. 1988. *Human Inquiry in Action*. London: Sage Publications.

Rogers, C.R. 1969. *Freedom to Learn – A View of What Education Might Become*. Columbus, OH: Charles Merrill.

Royal College of Nursing 1990. *Quality Patient Care: The Dynamic Standard Setting System*. Harrow, Middlesex: Scutari.

Schon, D.A. 1983. *The Reflective Practitioner: How Professionals Think in Action*. London: Temple Smith.

Schwarz, R. 2002. *The Skilled Facilitator*. San Francisco, CA: Jossey-Bass.

Stetler, C., Legro, M., Rycroft-Malone, J., Bowman, C., Curran, G., Guihan, M., et al. 2006. Role of 'external facilitation' in implementation of research findings: a qualitative evaluation of facilitation experiences in the Veterans Health Administration. *Implementation Science*, 1, 23.

Van de Ven, A.H. 2007. *Engaged Scholarship: A Guide to Organizational and Social Research*. Oxford: Oxford University Press.

Van de Ven, A.H., Pollet, D., Garud, R. & Venkataraman, S. 1999. *The Innovation Journey*. New York: Oxford University Press.

Yin, R.K. 2009. *Case Study Research: Design and Methods*. Thousand Oaks, CA: Sage.

6

FACILITATING AN EVIDENCE-BASED INNOVATION INTO PRACTICE

The novice facilitator's role

Alison Kitson and Gill Harvey

Introduction

In Chapter 4 we described a facilitation model that we have developed to operationalise the i-PARIHS framework. In Chapter 5, we then went on to outline a journey from starting out as a novice facilitator and moving to becoming an experienced or expert facilitator. In this chapter, our aim is to illustrate how a novice facilitator can begin to apply the facilitation model in practice. In the following chapter, we will continue this discussion, looking more specifically at the role of experienced and expert facilitators.

In describing the different facilitator roles, we noted that facilitators can be identified from within their local group, team, unit or organisation or they can be from another unit or organisation. These are referred to as internal and external facilitators, respectively. We also considered the sorts of people who become facilitators; what their personal qualities are and the skills and knowledge they need to help them become confident and accomplished facilitators. We compared other types of roles that are commonly used to help with the implementation of evidence into practice and suggested that these roles are necessary but not sufficient to achieve the whole task.

This chapter will concentrate on the basic building blocks for effective facilitation by describing a 'Facilitator's Toolkit' with the 'nuts and bolts' that are needed to engage local teams and individuals in the implementation process. Facilitators, whether they are internal or external to the organisation, should ideally be supported by experienced and expert facilitators. What is also important to note is that there are many different ways or routes to start the facilitation journey. Individuals may find themselves part of an organisation-wide project (as described by Elliott, 2014) where the timeframes and support for innovation have to be juggled against multiple other priorities. Alternatively, facilitators may be recruited to a research project, specifically designed to explore what facilitation is about (see the case study Chapters 8–12 for examples of this). Facilitators may be 'conscripted' into the role or they may 'volunteer'. They may be supported in a structured way by more experienced facilitators or they may find themselves alone and isolated, without proper guidance and support. All these scenarios happen and again, our objective is to help facilitators know what to do in such circumstances, so that they can get the best out of the situation.

We need to stress that facilitation should not be a lone activity. Ideally, the introduction of innovations or new evidence to a system is done in a planned, coordinated way, using the skills and talents of novice facilitators working under the direction and guidance of more experienced facilitators. These more experienced facilitators can either be internal or external to the organisation, depending on the size and scale of the project.

Starting out, the novice facilitator needs to become broadly familiar with some of the theories we presented in Chapter 3, for example, theories about the nature of innovations and how they relate to evidence appraisal and implementation. The next range of theories to be considered is around understanding what motivates individuals and teams to want to change what they do and how they work effectively together. These are considered in relation to the sort of environment or local contexts where people interact and work. At this stage less attention is paid to the wider contextual or organisational factors that influence what happens at a local level. The bulk of the learning focuses around what we call the basic skills of facilitation. This encompasses four dimensions within the Facilitator's Toolkit, described as: 'Clarify and engage', 'Assess and measure', 'Action and implementation' and finally, 'Review and share'.

Novice facilitators may be from outside of the organisation or area where the implementation is to occur. They may have done some local facilitation in the past; however, their experience in working in a new organisation or across organisations is limited, hence their novice status. Many implementation research projects use this type of external facilitator approach, as do some primary care prevention initiatives, where external facilitation models have proved quite successful (Baskerville et al., 2012). Important to that success is the support the novice external facilitators receive from the expert facilitation team.

The novice facilitator, as we described in Chapter 5, may already have experienced good or poor facilitation and it is from this experiential learning base that we can begin to build the theoretical understanding behind the many practical skills and tasks that become part of the Facilitator's Toolkit. The novice internal and external facilitators are provided with an

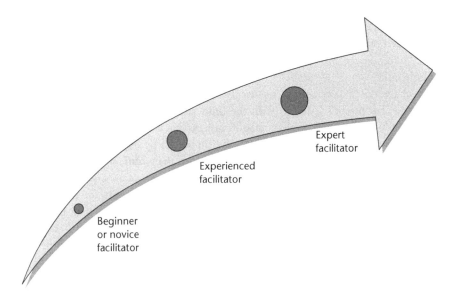

FIGURE 6.1 What do you need to know as a novice facilitator?

outline of how the different theories described in Chapter 3 integrate around the i-PARIHS framework and inform the Facilitator's Toolkit (Table 6.1). This includes:

- theories that help the facilitator understand what innovations are and how they relate to evidence-based practice approaches;
- theories that help understand how the recipients of innovation (individually and as a group or team) accept or adopt new knowledge;
- theories that help explain how the context or setting influences the way new knowledge is introduced and applied;
- theories that inform the practice of facilitation and help shape their own ability to work with individuals and teams to implement change.

We have described the main elements of each of these theories in Chapter 3 and would encourage you to refer back to this chapter if you want to remind yourself about the theories. The main focus of this chapter is to give you a set of practical tools and techniques that you can use to operationalise the i-PARIHS framework.

The Facilitator's Toolkit has emerged from a number of iterations where the contents have been tested as part of knowledge translation implementation studies. The first of these was in a project called TOPIC7 (Wiechula et al., 2009; Kitson et al., 2011), where the four phases were used to structure the way the facilitators worked with local implementation teams. A refined version of this approach was used in the Signature Project (see Chapter 12) and the refinements from the Signature and other work have been described in a Joanna Briggs Institute monograph (Kitson et al., 2012). The Toolkit, as it is presented in this chapter, is the result of several years' testing and refining. It has also incorporated the broader dimension of the i-PARIHS framework.

TABLE 6.1 Theories that underpin the Facilitator's Toolkit

Focus of facilitation	Relevant theories to consider
Innovation	<ul><li>Evidence-based decision-making</li><li>Experiential, problem-based and situated learning</li><li>Diffusion of innovations</li><li>Engaged scholarship</li></ul>
Recipients	<ul><li>Diffusion of innovations</li><li>Readiness to change</li><li>Theoretical domains framework</li><li>Communities of practice</li><li>Sticky knowledge and boundary theory</li></ul>
Context	<ul><li>Complexity/complex adaptive systems</li><li>Distributed leadership</li><li>Organisational culture</li><li>Learning organisation</li><li>Absorptive capacity</li><li>Sustainability</li></ul>
Facilitation	<ul><li>Humanist/student-centred learning</li><li>Cooperative inquiry</li><li>Quality improvement</li></ul>

There are four parts to the Facilitator's Toolkit (Figure 6.2). Each section or phase involves focused activities and there is a range of tools available to guide progression through each phase. We will describe the phases in a sequential way; however, in practice, there is likely to be a more iterative process, with overlap and movement between the different phases.

Phase 1: Clarify and engage

This phase involves determining the scope and focus of the project (Figure 6.3). It is an important engagement process that helps to locate the need for change at a local level. This involves the use of tools to first document all aspects of the issue of concern, identify specific problem areas and then prioritise the areas for targeted activity (Table 6.2).

We will briefly describe the key steps in this first phase.

Identify the issue of concern and key aspects related to it

One of the first tasks is to assess the need for new knowledge or to be able to estimate the 'gap' between the new knowledge and the actual way people are doing their jobs, whether they are frontline staff, educators or policy-makers. Justification for changing what we are doing can come from a wide range of areas, both formal and informal. Formal routes can be from quality improvement reports, safety reports or part of the strategic plan of the organisation, department or unit. Informal routes include responding to individual patient experiences or accounts or concerns voiced by members of staff or carers where little 'hard' data exists but there is a view that things are not right.

Importantly, the facilitator and the team leading the work need to convince other key stakeholders that the issue is worth spending time on and that improvements will benefit patient care, staff and the organisation. There are a number of simple checklists that can be used

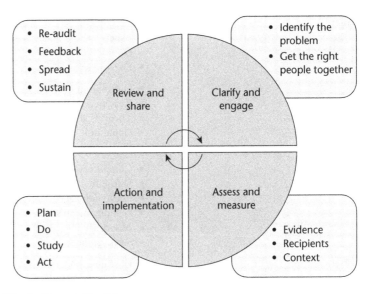

FIGURE 6.2 The Facilitator's Toolkit

TABLE 6.2 Elements of the 'clarify and engage' phase

Steps	Purpose
1. Identify with local stakeholders the problem, issue of concern	To establish how much commitment and interest there is in the topic. This will influence staff involvement and receptiveness to change
2. Identify members and bring a group together	To ascertain who the local champions are and what skills and knowledge are needed to create a group that has the capability to solve the problem and introduce the new knowledge
3. Refine the problem or issue of concern	Start with refining the problem to discrete time-limited elements that have evidence to support them and can be tackled in a practical way
4. Check what evidence exists related to the problem, issue of concern	Use the refined definition of the problem to access current evidence to determine if there is sufficient evidence to proceed with the topic, or if evidence needs to be generated locally
5. Produce a preliminary plan	This plan outlines the broad purpose of the project, identifies the expected benefits to patient care and staff experiences and outlines the expected resources required
6. Present to key stakeholders both at local level and at organisational level	The group shares the plan with key stakeholders in the organisation who need to support the work in order for it to be successful

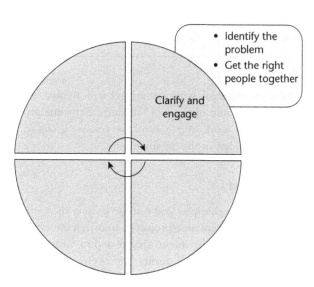

FIGURE 6.3 Phase 1: Clarify and engage

to organise these early conversations. For example, the set of questions given in Box 6.1 can be used to structure the first meeting you have with colleagues around a suggested improvement or innovation.

BOX 6.1   QUESTIONS TO FRAME A DISCUSSION AROUND THE INNOVATION

1.   What local data do you have that tells you that you have a problem?
2.   How reliable are the sources of data?
3.   What do your colleagues think about the problem?
4.   How are you currently managing the issue?
5.   What do your clients think about this?
6.   What research evidence exists about what best practice is?
7.   Describe what 'success' would look like if you addressed this problem

---

Organising a group

At this early planning stage it is really important to create a practical workable structure around the project. Support from your experienced or expert facilitator is invaluable. Establishing an implementation or project team is the next step (Box 6.2). You will need to ascertain that team members are interested in the topic to be investigated and it is always better to get volunteers rather than 'conscripts' (i.e. people who are forced to take part).

BOX 6.2   GETTING THE RIGHT TEAM TOGETHER

1.   Who needs to be on the team to make the project work?
2.   What skills do you need on the team?
3.   How are you going to get potential team members interested in the work?

Explain to the team members what the project will involve, make sure you organise regular meetings and put them into everyone's schedules. Set some ground rules and be clear about the way the group will work. Agree also how you are going to share your work with other colleagues and stakeholders in the organisation.

Refining the problem

There are a number of techniques you can use to help the team refine their topic. Often the real challenge with implementation projects is to match the evidence with an aspect of practice that is sufficiently discrete to be able to change and to measure that change. There are a number of techniques from the field of quality improvement and system redesign that can help to structure the group's prioritisation process, such as the use of an affinity diagram (a method to sort ideas and thoughts into groups with a common theme) or the 'fishbone' cause and effect tool (to organise the group's current knowledge regarding a problem or issue). Organisations such as the Institute for Healthcare Improvement (www.ihi.org) have useful information on their website about the different tools available and guidance on how to use them.

Check the evidence base of the proposed topic

It is important early on to check how much evidence exists on the proposed topic. It is advisable at this stage to access best practice guidelines, the Cochrane or Joanna Briggs Institute libraries of systematic reviews or any other sources of evidence available to inform your decision-making. Use the refined topic to help define the key words you can use to search online databases. One of the first jobs of the newly created project team is then to read through the existing evidence to see how much there is, how relevant it is and how it might be used. You can use this step to involve your team in talking about the evidence and encourage them to think in different ways about their own practice.

Produce a preliminary plan

It is helpful even at this early stage to set out what you propose to do in a systematic way. Outline your project aims in relation to your initial topic area, your broad objectives, and the proposed timeframe you are working within. This is the project plan you will be working with over the next few weeks or months and as you go through each of the phases of the Toolkit you will be able to refine and alter it. Importantly, you should try at this stage to define what 'success' would look like, both in terms of patient care, but also in relation to the way staff work together and their working practices and culture. You will be able to refine these areas after you have gone through the 'Assess and measure' phase of the Toolkit.

Present the project plan to stakeholders at a local and organisational level

Before any detailed work starts, it is advisable, with help from the experienced or expert facilitator who is supporting you to organise a session for key stakeholders. This is to ensure that there is wider support and a shared understanding about the project, that people are clear who is involved and what the benefits are to the organisation. It is also a good idea to develop a project communications plan at this early stage. Minimally you should keep your stakeholders and your team members updated with progress. Finally, try to put a timeframe round the work and, as far as possible, stick to it.

Phase 2: Assess and measure

As the facilitator, you should now be at a point where you have identified and refined your topic and assembled a team of willing colleagues with whom to work. The topic is the innovation (i.e. it becomes the new piece of evidence that will be introduced to practice). Importantly, the 'assess and measure' phase involves understanding how the underlying evidence (from guidelines, clinical experience, patient preferences and local data) informing the innovation can be transformed into local standards or goals for improvement (Figure 6.4). From here the new knowledge can be developed into local measurement criteria that can be compared against current practice. These criteria are compiled into an audit tool and used to undertake a baseline audit.

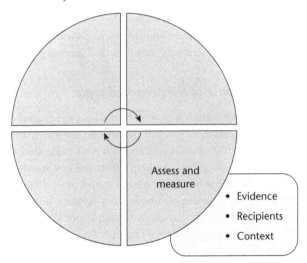

FIGURE 6.4 Phase 2: Assess and measure

As well as getting the evidence informing the innovation together, this phase helps the facilitator and the project team to begin to understand the other factors that will need to be addressed if the implementation process is going to succeed. This includes assessing and measuring how individuals and teams (the recipients) are going to respond to the innovation and what impact the local and organisational context will have (inner context).

There are three steps to this phase (understanding evidence, understanding the recipients and understanding context) and they help to create a deeper understanding of the multiple factors at play in trying to introduce new ideas into practice (Table 6.3).

Understanding evidence

The novice facilitator, by this stage, will have worked with their local project team to outline the potential topic and will have looked at the literature to get some sense of the research evidence informing the subject. However, what they will not have done at this first stage is to look in detail at the wider types of evidence that also inform the innovation. This is what they will now do with their team.

There are three main things to consider: the nature of the evidence, how it is 'packaged' and how likely it is to be accepted or contested by those people who have to implement it. Table 6.4 outlines these main areas together with the skills needed by the facilitator to actively shape the team's activity.

The facilitator guides the team through the process, identifying appropriate clinical guidelines, determining agreed standards or goals, determining measurement criteria and translating these criteria into an audit tool. These elements are evidence-based but also are specific for the context in which you are measuring practice.

TABLE 6.3 Elements of the 'assess and measure' phase

Steps	Purpose
1. Understanding evidence	• Familiarisation with the different types of evidence • From evidence to local standards or goals for improvement • Developing and applying a local audit tool with measurement criteria
2. Understanding the recipients	• How to motivate individuals • How to get and keep a group working effectively
3. Understanding context	• Familiarisation with the different aspects and influences of context • From broad understanding of context to local interpretation of the barriers and enablers to successful implementation • How to develop or apply a local context assessment tool

TABLE 6.4 Assessing the characteristics of the evidence

Characteristics of the evidence	Facilitator skill and knowledge
What is the underlying evidence for the proposed innovation or change? Is it derived from research? Is it based on clinical consensus? Is it informed by robust ways of collecting patient experiences? Does it use data from local audits?	Acquiring and appraising the evidence
Is the evidence 'packaged' in an accessible and usable form (e.g. a clinical guideline, a care pathway, an algorithm)? How much adaptation of the information will be required to make it manageable for implementation at local level? Does it come with a set of measurable criteria or will these have to be developed?	Developing local standards and aims for improvement from larger evidence-based guidelines Developing local audits that can be used to measure baseline activity and re-audit post implementation
Is the evidence likely to be controversial? Is there a shared view about the rigour and importance? How likely is it to be accepted or challenged by those people who have to implement it? Can it be tested out with a small group before formal implementation?	Preliminary testing through discussion in phase 1 Plan–Do–Study–Act (PDSA) methods

Understanding recipients

In addition to the more technical work around the evidence, the novice facilitator has the opportunity to assess the level of motivation and interest in the innovation at an individual and collective level. Questions such as those listed in Table 6.5 can be used to help the facilitator gauge the receptiveness to the innovation and devise strategies to influence the attitudes and behaviour of the recipients.

TABLE 6.5 Assessing the characteristics of the recipients

The recipients of the innovation	Facilitator skill and knowledge
Are people motivated to introduce the innovation at an individual and collective level? Do they want to apply it in practice?	Engaging and motivating colleagues
Is the proposed change seen as valuable? Will everyone see a need to make a change? Is there a shared view or are there differences of opinion between key individuals or between different professional groups?	Consensus building methods
Are there existing data that can be used to highlight the potential for improvement?	Audit and feedback
Are there clinical champions supporting the change?	Agreeing shared goals
Are people able to implement the proposed change at an individual and collective level?	Project management including resource planning
Do they understand what the change entails? Is it within their current level of knowledge and skills? Do people understand the modifications that will be needed to routine practice and how to change and embed these?	Visioning and sense making
Will additional training and development be needed? Are the resources available to support the implementation process? Do people feel they have the necessary authority to carry out the proposed changes?	Liaising and negotiating with managers
Have key individuals/stakeholders whose support is needed been identified?	Identifying and engaging key stakeholders and opinion leaders
Are the potential barriers to implementation identified and discussed?	Identifying, assessing and managing boundary issues
Is there good inter-professional collaboration and teamwork – between professional groups and between clinical staff and managers?	Team building and collaborative working

What is important at this stage is for the facilitator to be able to assess the level of individual and collective engagement. As described in the first step (clarify and engage), the initial conversations with key stakeholders will have already begun. But it will be at this second step that a more formal assessment is carried out. This could include using a framework to structure the assessment, such as the Theoretical Domains Framework that was discussed in Chapter 3.

Understanding context

The novice facilitator and the project team consider the inner context in two ways: first, by assessing the immediate local context and then the wider departmental or organisational context. The primary concern of the novice facilitator tends to be on the inner context, while the outer context elements are the priority of experienced or expert facilitators guiding and supporting the novice facilitator and their team.

It makes sense to start off by looking at the immediate context in which the innovation is to be introduced (Table 6.6). For example, if the facilitator is working in a nursing home, then the context is the whole nursing home facility. But if the nursing home facility had many floors and the innovation was focusing on just one of these floors, then the initial assessment of context would be for that floor only. However, this does not mean that external contextual factors do not also influence the local context.

TABLE 6.6 Assessing the characteristics of the inner local context

The inner context: local level	Facilitator skill and knowledge
Infrastructure and resources	
Is there sufficient time to undertake the project at local level?	Organisation context
Are staff able to get involved?	assessment
Is there a commitment to provide the right financial resources?	
Is the infrastructure including equipment and electronic communications able to cope with the proposed changes?	
Are there any perceived structural (fitness of purpose of the buildings and environment) challenges?	
Are the any systems (patient administration, workflow, management, safety and quality systems) challenges?	
Culture	
What are the prevailing values and beliefs of the local context where the innovation is being introduced?	Assessment of culture
How involved do individuals feel in change?	
Are individual's roles and responsibilities clearly understood?	
How do individuals at local level describe the culture?	
Do patients and staff feel valued?	
Is there a culture that supports innovation and change?	
Leadership	
Who are the formal and informal leaders at local level?	Getting a sense of who the
Are they likely to be supportive of the proposed change?	formal and informal leaders
Are the leaders helping to create a facilitative context through providing motivation and support, creating a vision and reinforcing the change process?	are and how they can be involved
Do leaders support individual staff members to take on new roles?	
Do teams work effectively?	
Can individuals and teams make decisions effectively?	
Is leadership distributed or more hierarchical?	
Learning and evaluation	
Are there mechanisms in place for staff to receive feedback on their work (regular team meetings, audit and feedback processes, professional development opportunities and performance review systems)?	Assessing openness and receptiveness to using new knowledge to shape decisions and actions
Is there any experience of involvement in external evaluation or organisation-wide audits at local level?	
What is the past experience of introducing change?	
Is there evidence of a learning culture?	

It is also useful to think about how the proposed innovation at a local level will be supported at a wider organisational level (Table 6.7). This is an area where the input of a more experienced facilitator is helpful in terms of guiding the novice facilitator and highlighting the key factors to look out for.

Assessing and managing the local context is essential for successful implementation. Applying the sorts of questions listed in Tables 6.6 and 6.7 helps the facilitator and the team to anticipate and plan how they manage their resources, negotiate the right sort of leadership support, shape the culture and create effective learning mechanisms to embed and sustain the innovation. To supplement this initial assessment, they may also elect to use some of the formal context assessment measures that we described in chapter four. Importantly, the facilitator aims to distinguish between those contextual factors which directly impact at a local level and those that have to be addressed at the wider organisational level. The role of the novice facilitator is very much to assess and manage the local context and to work with the experienced or expert facilitator in understanding and addressing the wider organisational context.

TABLE 6.7 Assessing the characteristics of the inner organisational context

The inner context: organisational level	Facilitator skill and knowledge
Infrastructure and resources	
Do the evidence/innovation and the changes proposed align with the strategic priorities for the organisation?	Assessment undertaken in collaboration with the experienced or expert facilitator and a plan developed
Does the organisation have systems and processes in place that support innovation and change (e.g. effective information and communication systems, opportunities for networking and learning across departments/teams)?	
Are there mechanisms in place for embedding changes in routine practice (e.g. formal policies and procedures)?	
Culture	
Is there a culture that supports innovation and change across the whole organisation?	Implementation may happen at local level but stall at organisational level because of the wider cultural factors – important to anticipate possible areas of challenge and start conversations early
Is there a history of successful and sustained change within the organisation?	
Are the organisational values and philosophy clear?	
Do the espoused values reflect how the organisation functions?	
Leadership	
Does the senior leadership team of the organisation actively seek opportunities for improvement/innovation by involving consumers, the public and staff?	Assessing the level of commitment and capacity of leaders to embrace and champion change. Working with them to identify 'quick wins' and opportunities
Do senior leaders actively engage with local staff?	
Learning and evaluation	
Are there robust organisation-wide feedback mechanisms to provide staff with credible feedback on their performance?	Understanding the importance of providing feedback on the project and using existing systems and processes to build up new routines
Is the organisation receptive to new knowledge?	
Is there evidence of absorptive capacity?	

Phase 3: Action and implementation

The 'assess and measure' phase has been about getting ready for action and implementation. The novice facilitator and their team will have undertaken a baseline audit or assessment of existing practice related to the topic of interest. Once performance levels are established through the audit process this next phase involves the use of tools to plan and implement appropriate strategies to improve performance. These methods draw heavily on quality improvement approaches (such as Plan–Do–Study–Act – or PDSA cycles) as well as learning principles derived from action science, learning organisations and communities of practice (Figure 6.5).

This period represents a mix of 'hard' and 'soft' approaches to experiential learning. For example, in addition to the baseline audit, there will be information about recipients' readiness to change and data on the local context and what needs to be done to prepare it for the proposed change.

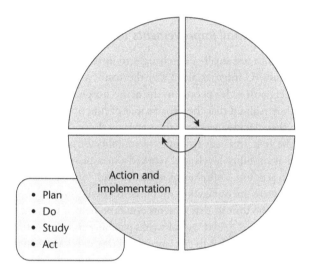

FIGURE 6.5 Phase 3: Action and implementation

TABLE 6.8 Elements of the 'action and implementation' phase

Steps	Purpose
1. Interpretation of baseline data and creation of an action plan	Ensuring that everyone involved in the implementation knows what their current practice is and understand the need to change
2. Identify, introduce and test the impact of small improvements	Prioritise actions and agree how to do it. Undertake first PDSA cycle
3. Proceed with introduction of planned changes using group to monitor progress	Use repeat PDSA cycles to build up a picture of where and how change should happen and where there are pockets of resistance
4. Agree timeframe for the implementation process and set final post-implementation audit/chart review	Structured approach to introducing new knowledge, processes and skills enables the team to understand what is happening

Interpretation of baseline audit, recipient and contextual readiness for change

From the results of the audit the project team will know what aspects of practice need to change and what is working according to best practice. In addition, the facilitator will have collected information about what individuals and teams think of the change, how they are motivated to get involved and how conducive the organisation is to support any changes. These different types of data – the clinical, the motivational and behavioural and the organisational and contextual – come together to create the plan of action.

Often analysis and interpretation of the audit findings happens simultaneously and clinical staff immediately want to change things. However, one of the jobs of the facilitator is to encourage the team to think about the implementation plan in a structured way and in particular consider the behavioural and contextual factors that, if not addressed, will reduce the chance of long-term success.

Identify and test small improvements using PDSA cycles

It is always good to test small-scale changes to introduce improvements in practice. For example, in one study (Gordge et al., 2009) the team wanted to look at how they could reduce functional decline in older people in the acute hospital setting. Having looked at the relevant guidelines, they realised that the broad topic of functional decline was much too big for them to handle so they decided to break their activity down by looking at one area of improvement at a time. The first area was to improve mobility of patients in the orthopaedic unit, so the team looked at mobility levels and worked out a plan of how they could improve this. The plan took into account a number of structural and contextual issues at unit level. For example, when patients were encouraged to mobilise following surgery the ward team decided to set up a dining area in the unit so that patients could be helped to walk there to have lunch.

This small change required several weeks planning and negotiation and the local facilitators had to work with all stakeholders to convince them this additional activity was worth the effort. They had to engage safety and risk personnel to get support for mobilising patients and they also had to work with the catering department to ensure that patients' lunches were brought to the correct place on the ward. In addition, nursing and physiotherapy staff had to work together to agree best practice around mobilising certain patients. So, what seemed to be a relatively straightforward idea – to encourage patients to mobilise in order to reduce the risk of functional decline – became quite a complex change-management process involving many different actors in the system.

The PDSA cycle

The PDSA cycle helps the project team to structure their actions, predict whether or not they will work as planned, then test and evaluate the changes and refine them accordingly. Table 6.9 illustrates the use of the PDSA approach with the above mobilisation example (Gordge et al., 2009).

Why test change?

The above example illustrates how even a very obvious improvement in a routine practice (mobilising fractured neck of femur patients to reduce the risk of functional decline) is

TABLE 6.9 An example of applying a PDSA cycle

Plan	
Objective	Audit data showed that older patients were not being mobilised routinely according to best practice guidelines
	Objective was to test how to increase mobilisation of fractured neck of femur patients post operatively in one orthopaedic ward
Predictions	Nurses would say they were too busy to undertake this activity
	Physiotherapists would say it was not their responsibility
	Safety and quality department would be concerned about increased risk of falls
Develop the test (who, what, when, where)	The team needed to come up with a way of mobilising patients that was not perceived to be increasing nurses' workload, that was safe and that added to the recovery of patients
	The test was to see whether a small number of patients (2 to begin with) could be helped to walk down to a day room (a converted store room) in order to have lunch. This would involve the nursing and physiotherapy staff assessing risk and agreeing a method of supporting mobilisation, preparing the room and liaising with catering staff
Do	
Try out the test on a small scale	Two patients were selected on the first day
Observe and document	Staff and patients were asked to give feedback. Consideration was given to how to measure the amount of mobilisation undertaken
Study	
Analyse data	Following the pilot the team increased the number of patients walking to the dining room
Study the results	Data were collected at the end of an agreed time period that looked at level of mobilisation and staff and patient responses
Compare, summarise and reflect	The intervention showed mobility for this subgroup of patients had improved and that levels of satisfaction were high from both patients and staff
Act	
Refine, modify	The challenge facing the team however, was how to spread the initiative beyond a few patients and how to create a more permanent and appropriate dining area for patients
Prepare for next cycle	During the time that the team were preparing for this, nursing staffing levels on the unit were affected by winter pressures and sickness and the team had to hold off its next cycle of activity

multi-layered and complex. It required the cooperation and support of several departments and professional groups in the organisation and even when the preliminary testing proved positive it was still difficult to embed into practice because of resource issues.

Despite these real challenges, what is important about taking a structured approach is that the team has evidence to show colleagues. This increases belief about the usefulness of the new activity and it documents expectations of different stakeholders. Undertaking a series of PDSA cycles builds a common understanding and it can also evaluate and record costs and any unintended side effects.

More sophisticated use of PDSA cycles can help to explore theories in a predictive way. For example, one of the observations from the mobilisation study was that patients not only benefitted from walking to the dining room but also chatted more and ate more food. Such clinical observations could be enhanced by testing this approach out over a longer term to see whether addressing some of the structural aspects of context (e.g. whether dining rooms should be a option for wards with high numbers of immobile and dependent older patients) could improve care. Involving frontline staff in such tests creates a commitment to improvement and innovation.

Repeated use of PDSA cycles will result in changes that lead to improvement, but it may take many cycles. You can start off with a hunch or a theory, you can test it, and you can learn from the failures of that test. Working with the implementation project team, you can undertake multiple small-scale tests, adapting your approach based on what you learned from the previous test. When you are reaching a high level of achievement in the small-scale setting, you can then test it over a broader area (e.g. perhaps over the whole ward rather than one bay or in two or three different clinical settings) and if that is successful you may choose to scale up even further. Eventually, when you have tested multiple cycles, over different time periods and across different settings, you should feel that it is sufficiently robust to be offered as a change to other areas that are interested in the innovation.

Introduction of planned changes

The repeat PDSA cycles will start to build up a picture of where the local context will be supportive of the proposed changes and where progress will be more challenging. The findings from the local context assessment will also help the team to interpret why certain things do not go according to plan. Likely barriers to change can be considered and then small PDSA cycles can be introduced to test a particular approach.

Most change requires shifts in attitudes, knowledge, skills and behaviour. This means that most changes will require some sort of education or coaching of staff and/or patients. Often PDSA cycles will include the introduction of new educational material to staff in order to develop knowledge, skills and the capacity to change.

Final post-implementation audit

The last step in the 'action and implementation' phase is to agree on the timeframe for the implementation phase proper and decide when the final audit will be undertaken. By this time the team and the facilitator(s) will have gone through a number of pilot and repeat PDSA cycles, each reflecting an important dimension of the evidence-based innovation they want to implement. It is important to keep commitment and interest in the project going as there is nothing worse than projects going on for months without any real progress. It is important for the novice facilitator and the team to keep key stakeholders updated about progress and to seek help and support from them as needed to address some of the more complex context or resource-related challenges.

Setting a finish date is always good at the start of any project. It can be renegotiated but at least it sets the parameters for the facilitator and the team to plan the work. Also, once a project team has experienced the implementation cycle within the Toolkit, they will be able to look at other areas of improvement.

The 'action and implementation' phase is a busy and exciting time. It requires focused planning and communication with all stakeholders. The important thing is not to try to do too much at the beginning. Once the audit results have given you baseline data, you need to break down your plan into 'bite-size chunks' of change. Go for small improvements that have the support of staff and that are not too labour intensive or controversial. Keep everyone engaged and involved and when you run into your first challenge bring the team together to creatively problem solve.

By following the above steps you should be able to understand which contextual factors will support your implementation strategy and which will require further work. Remember to keep your stakeholders on side and recruit the support of colleagues with educational and coaching skills. Many improvements require new knowledge and skills development. And most importantly, remember change always takes longer than you think, but despite this still set some deadlines in order to keep colleagues involved and engaged.

Phase 4: Review and share

The last phase of any implementation project involves reviewing the action phase to determine if improvements have occurred (Figure 6.6). This analysis will determine if new cycles need to be undertaken or if a repeat cycle is required for further improvement. It is important to share the results of the project, not just to all those involved but more broadly to build the knowledge base around implementing evidence-based innovation. Table 6.10 details some of the activities to be undertaken in this phase.

Collecting evidence of improvement using clinical, recipient and contextual sources of data

The results of the post-implementation audit should be shared with all those involved in the project. In addition to the clinical audit data, it is important to discuss some of the wider

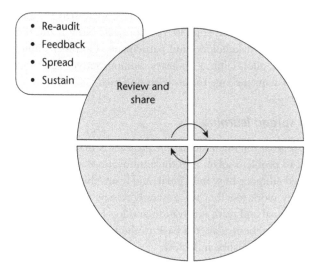

FIGURE 6.6 Phase 4: Review and share

TABLE 6.10 Elements of the 'review and share' phase

Step	Purpose
1. Collect any evidence of improvement – using clinical audit, contextual and staff data	To check that planned improvement using the new knowledge along with the methods of facilitating its introduction into the clinical setting has worked (or not)
2. Guided reflection on what worked well and what did not go to plan	To learn from the experience and to share that learning in a constructive, informed way
3. Feedback to stakeholders	To close off the project and to inform the stakeholders what worked, how things have improved, what learning occurred and what the next actions are
4. Plans for building on the work and spreading the learning	Review of next steps and how to sustain the improvement
5. Organising a 'celebratory event' and publication	To symbolise the end of the project and to celebrate the success
6. Assess capacity development and potential or ongoing partnerships between key stakeholders	Review benefits of establishing partnerships with different teams or groups that were involved in the project. Review how the facilitation process worked and what the novice, experienced and expert facilitators learnt

individual and team, contextual, process and organisational factors that may have impeded or enabled the successful implementation of the evidence. Even if the results were not as far reaching as hoped, often the lessons learnt from things not going to plan are as important as the successes. Make sure that everyone feels valued and appreciated for their efforts and plan how you want to share your achievements.

Feedback to stakeholders

At the beginning of the project you will have identified the range of key stakeholders that needed to know about and support your project. Now is the time to complete a report and distribute it to key stakeholders and participants. Consider different stakeholder groups such as patients, colleagues, clinical, industry, administrative, educational and legislative decision-makers. Tailor your message to suit their interests.

Build and spread learning

The ultimate goal for implementation projects is that they become part of the way clinical teams work to problem solve, introduce innovations and improve care. The skills and knowledge acquired embrace how individuals and teams think about the evidence base of their practice, how they work together to constantly review and improve their practice, and how they manage individual and team motivation and local contexts. It is important, therefore, that the project team's experiences are fed back to the leaders in the organisation who set the strategic goals and targets for quality and safety.

Most importantly, you do not want to lose the skills and knowledge gained through facilitating an implementation project team. Equally, any practice improvements made in one area need to be spread to other areas. This may be where you might want to explore such things as communities of practice or virtual learning networks. Having a forum where staff can come together to talk about their practice is a very powerful mechanism for change. Although some organisations would not consider this special, for many professional groups, such as nurses, opportunities to come together to discuss clinical issues are limited. Facilitation of these types of meetings can be an effective way to promote learning and knowledge sharing.

The celebratory event

Organising a 'celebratory event' is an important milestone in the project. It symbolises the end of the implementation cycle and is an opportunity for all those involved to share their experiences – celebrating the successes and learning from what did not go as planned. A celebratory event can be a group presentation in the unit followed by coffee and cakes or it can be a conference with invited speakers and leaders who can be influenced by the presentations. It is up to the facilitator and the team to decide how they want to use the event to shape future activity. In particular the event acknowledges the work and commitment of the facilitators and the implementation team and encourages others to be involved in future activity.

Assess capacity development and partnerships

By the time the novice facilitator and the team have reached this point, they will have a clear understanding of what has worked, what needed more attention or support and what did not need to be done. This reflective and evaluative step involves the experienced and expert facilitators debriefing with the novice facilitator and the team. Depending on the size and scale of the project, there may be just one novice facilitator and one more experienced facilitator having a chat over a cup of coffee to debrief or it may involve several novice facilitators working with teams across multiple sites mentored and supported by a team of experienced and expert facilitators. In the case studies, there are examples of implementation projects over multiple sites (Chapters 8, 9, 10 and 12) and those that focused in one organisation (Chapter 11).

This debriefing will help the organisation decide how it wishes to invest in building facilitation capacity for future innovation and implementation initiatives. Creating a network of expert and experienced facilitators (for example, located in academic or health service research and development departments specialising in innovation, knowledge translation, implementation and improvement science or evaluation) working in partnership with healthcare staff and organisations also enables stronger links between research and practice. This model is at the heart of what Van de Ven (2007) calls engaged scholarship, where researchers and practitioners work together on complex and challenging problems. The strategic goals of both academic and healthcare organisations need to embrace this sort of dynamic interaction in order to capitalize and build on the organisational investment in facilitation. Organisational models such as Academic Health Science Centres and Networks build on this notion but to date have tended to focus on more linear, 'pipeline' models of knowledge translation rather than a more interactive and facilitative approach. There is a real opportunity to reshape this agenda.

Summary/conclusion

In this chapter we have described how facilitators can begin to shape the introduction of an innovation into practice. Supported by a number of explicit theories and practical steps, novice facilitators are mentored by more experienced facilitators. By following the phases of the Facilitator's Toolkit, novice facilitators can gain confidence in managing the multi-dimensionality and complexity of change. In our next chapter we outline what the key roles of more experienced and expert facilitators are and how they can optimise the sustainability and spread of innovations across the organisation.

References

Baskerville, N.B., Liddy, C. & Hogg, W. 2012. Systematic review and meta-analysis of practice facilitation within primary care settings. *Annals of Family Medicine*, 10, 63–74.

Elliott, J. 2014. How does an acute care setting respond to a national directive in introducing an organizational wide innovation? A descriptive single case study. Master of Nursing Science, University of Adelaide.

Gordge, L., De Young, J. & Wiechula, R. 2009. Reducing functional decline of older people in an acute-care setting: are we providing adequate care to maintain/optimise the functional status of our elder patients? *International Journal of Evidence Based Healthcare*, 7, 181–6.

Kitson, A., Wiechula, R., Zeitz, K., Marcionni, D., Page, T. & Silverston, H. 2011. Improving older peoples' care in one acute hospital setting: a realist evaluation of a KT intervention. Adelaide: University of Adelaide.

Kitson, A., Wiechula, R., Salmond, S. & Jordan, Z. 2012. *Knowledge Translation in Healthcare*. Philadelphia, PA: Lippincott Williams and Wilkins.

Van de Ven, A.H. 2007. *Engaged Scholarship: A Guide to Organizational and Social Research*. Oxford: Oxford University Press.

Wiechula, R., Kitson, A., Marcoionni, D., Page, T., Zeitz, K. & Silverston, H. 2009. Improving the fundamentals of care for older people in the acute hospital setting: facilitating practice improvement using a Knowledge Translation Toolkit. *International Journal of Evidence-Based Healthcare*, 7, 283–95.

7

DEVELOPING CAPACITY AND DRIVING THE SUSTAINABILITY AND SPREAD OF EVIDENCE-BASED INNOVATIONS

Alison Kitson and Gill Harvey

Introduction

In the i-PARIHS framework, we argue that facilitation is the driving force for the successful implementation of evidence-based innovation in practice. Facilitation is also an enabler for the successful embedding, sustaining and spread of the innovation across, within and between individuals, teams and organisations. Facilitation achieves this by focusing on relationships, individual and group learning and managing the myriad of contextual factors that make each implementation journey unique.

In Chapter 6 we outlined how novice facilitators can begin to develop their skill and expertise. In order to do this we have argued that they need support and guidance from more experienced or expert facilitators. In this chapter we will outline what we believe are the key attributes of experienced facilitation roles. These roles are often implicit in organisations and individuals with such skills may be involved in organisational development, change management, quality improvement and safety or educational and development activities.

We suggest that by making facilitation a more central element within these sort of roles, organisations will be able to harness more effective translation of new ideas into practice. They will have a more integrated strategic approach to how they are going to keep staff motivated, interested and curious to try out new ideas in a systematic, structured way. Our proposed solution is to create a more visible and structured network of experienced and expert facilitators who work in partnership between healthcare organisations and academic institutions focusing directly upon the 'science' of implementation and knowledge translation.

These roles would be jointly 'owned' by both organisations and would work to identify and develop novice facilitators who could learn on the job. As a result, the novice facilitators would learn how to develop more advanced facilitation skills and in turn could develop into experienced and expert facilitators. In Chapter 5 we outlined the key attributes of the three different levels of facilitation. Table 7.1 summarises the characteristics and skills that we think are required by experienced and expert facilitators.

Before we describe the roles it may be useful to say something about internal and external facilitation roles. We touched on this in an earlier chapter and described how facilitators can

TABLE 7.1 Characteristics and skills required by experienced and expert facilitators

Experienced facilitator	• Working under the supervision of an expert facilitator
	• In-depth understanding and knowledge of the organisation or organisations they are working with
	• Awareness of competing tensions and how to manage these around innovations
	• In-depth understanding of individual motivations and productivity
	• Knowledge of team motivation and productivity
	• Experienced and knowledgeable in local context evaluation
	• Able to assess system-wide activities and influence actions
	• Aware of wider contextual issues and confident in terms of managing boundaries and political tensions
	• Advanced skills of facilitation around the four phases of the Facilitator's Toolkit: clarify and engage; assess and measure; action and implementation; review and share
Expert facilitator	• Expert facilitator operating as a guide and mentor to other facilitators
	• Mentoring and coaching experienced facilitators
	• Coordinating facilitation networks
	• Working with systems to improve implementation success
	• Working across academic, service and other organisational boundaries to integrate facilitation and research activity
	• Developing and testing theories of implementation, innovation and facilitation
	• Evaluating interventions
	• Generating new knowledge
	• Refining and improving learning materials and mentoring processes
	• Running workshops and advanced master classes on facilitation approaches

belong to the organisation where they will be facilitating the change or they can come from the outside. There are advantages and disadvantages to either role. Importantly, it is likely that the more experienced and expert the facilitator, the more they will work with and in other organisations. Knox et al. (2011) have outlined the pros and cons of internal and external facilitation within primary care settings (Table 7.2) and this is consistent with facilitation roles in other types of healthcare system.

These pressures exist for any facilitator, whatever the level of experience. Again, it is important to set up a support network around facilitators to ensure they can get the most out of their activity.

The experienced facilitator: getting to grips with capacity development, mentoring and sustaining change

The experienced facilitator will have worked as a novice facilitator for a period of months, learning the skills and techniques of successful facilitation. Following the completion of a number of implementation projects, the novice facilitator should have developed the skills and confidence to lead larger implementation projects within or across organisations. Working under the supervision of an expert facilitator, they begin to develop their understanding of what it is like to take on a broader facilitation role. Here, the experienced facilitator assumes responsibility for mentoring and supporting the work of the novice facilitators, helping to problem-solve and deal with difficult or more challenging situations. Often these come in the

TABLE 7.2 Advantages and disadvantages of different types of facilitators

Type of facilitator	Advantages	Disadvantages
Internal to the practice or health system	Understands the culture, current processes, and personalities Likely to take ownership of the innovation more quickly	Often subject to a top-down approach More directly affected by internal politics, organisational pressures, and interpersonal dynamics Prone to being pulled into clinical care or other practice priorities (clinical demands outweigh the innovation)
External to the practice and health system	More likely to empower the practice and facilitate, rather than 'do for' the practice Clearer boundaries of roles Less likely to be affected by health system pressures	Can take longer to establish rapport and trust with practice and set expectations and goals Prone to becoming a crutch for the practice; might require tapering off of activities by facilitator

Source: After Knox et al. (2011).

guise of having to manage competing tensions around innovations; dealing with individual motivation and productivity in more complex circumstances; developing and extending the range of ways to optimise team motivation and productivity and paying ongoing and careful attention to the local context.

The experienced facilitation role also has the capacity to monitor and assess wider system activities and put into place actions that protect any local improvement and enable it to start to spread. The advanced skills of facilitation, based on the same theoretical domains as before, also encompass the four phases of clarifying and engaging with stakeholders, assessing and measuring, taking action and implementing the innovation and finally, reviewing and sharing the results. Importantly, the experienced facilitator brings to these an increased skill and knowledge base, for example, in terms of a more rigorous approach to the monitoring and evaluation of local initiatives, which can provide feedback to the local teams as evidence of their effectiveness.

We saw in previous chapters that many healthcare professionals possess a range of facilitation skills. Often, through experience or exposure to a quality improvement initiative or a research project, individuals may decide they want to have a more formal introduction to facilitation. They may volunteer to be part of an improvement project and through this are supported and mentored by a more experienced or expert facilitator. The case study chapters outline a number of scenarios where novice facilitators (from a wide variety of backgrounds and experiences) learnt how to be effective facilitators of practice improvement. These individuals would then be ready to take on further projects as experienced facilitators.

One example of how novice facilitators became more experienced facilitators was through a series of improvement projects undertaken in one large metropolitan hospital in South Australia (Wiechula et al., 2009; Kitson et al., 2011). In 2008 a project was set up to improve the experience of older people going through the acute hospital setting. Seven areas for improvement were identified across the hospital and two novice facilitators per topic were trained in the basic tools and techniques of the Facilitator's Toolkit. More experienced facilitators, in the role of project coordinators, supported each pair of novice facilitators and over a 12-month period the co-facilitators with their teams went through each of the stages outlined in the Toolkit. The results of the study showed that some progress was made in four of the seven areas and the evaluation was able to identify why this was the case (Gordge et al., 2009; McLeish et al., 2009; Wiechula et al., 2009; Kitson et al., 2010).

Following the completion of the study, one of the teams, which was looking at improving the nutritional experience of older people in hospital, decided it wanted to continue with its work. In collaboration with the research team and expert facilitator, the team gained support from the hospital executive group to fund a hospital-wide implementation of the best evidence around nutritional screening and practice. This project became the Prevention and Reduction of Weight Loss (PRoWL) project (see Chapter 11 for a more detailed description of the project). It involved the introduction of three linked interventions (universal nutritional screening; provision of nutritional fluids for those at risk; and assistance with eating and drinking) to reduce weight loss in vulnerable older people.

The novice facilitators from the original study were then paired with clinical staff who had undertaken a Joanna Briggs Institute Clinical Fellowships programme (http://joannabriggs. org/jbi-education.html). This project also brought together nurses and dieticians as co-facilitators. The approach used to introduce the system-wide intervention was found to be more successful than the earlier project and this was in part due to the enhanced experience and confidence of the facilitators.

The experienced facilitators who worked on the PRoWL project identified three important dimensions for developing capacity and sustaining change. The first of these was the importance of embedding the new evidence or ideas into the routines or habits of the nursing teams and catering staff. The experienced facilitators described how part of the challenge was to ensure that nutritional screening was undertaken as a standard part of the admission process, together with nursing staff asking questions about feeding assistance. Another routine was to target Sundays as 'weigh days'. This ensured that all patients' weights were up to date and accurate. Additionally, the process of monitoring 'at-risk' patients needing feeding assistance necessitated the catering staff and nursing teams introducing a 'red tray' system, in which nurses identified at-risk patients, who then received their food on a red tray. Important in managing this process was the fact that all parties involved understood what the red trays meant and they ensured they worked.

A second dimension was promoting a positive attitude about the innovation in all staff. In this example, the challenge was to encourage nursing staff to see nutrition as an important nursing responsibility in the myriad of tasks that had to be undertaken in a busy ward environment. This was tackled in a number of ways: addressing the importance of patient-centred care and meeting patients' fundamental care needs; providing evidence of the impact of neglecting this; looking at how the different services – catering, dietetics, stores and nursing – could work more collaboratively on this service improvement. The third dimension was the importance of introducing audit and feedback processes into the units so that staff could see what difference they were making.

Factors such as the three dimensions identified in the PRoWL project have been highlighted by other researchers looking at issues of capacity and sustainability. For example, the Normalisation Process Theory proposed by May and Finch (2009) illustrates the importance of new ideas finding their way into everyday routines through processes of building coherence and cognition, sense-making and collective action and monitoring, so that the innovation can be sustained. Kislov et al. (2014) also discuss the importance of capacity development being focused upon enhancing the capabilities and skills of individuals, groups and the organisation. They identify a need to develop first-, second- and third-order capabilities, First-order capabilities relate to the task in hand – understanding the problem, analysing the data and getting to grips with the evidence. Second-order capabilities relate to embracing improvement methodologies, while third-order capability links to the ability to transfer learning across teams and departments.

It was certainly evident from the PRoWL project that the facilitators were actively engaging with the staff in pro-active, supportive ways, building on the new routines, new attitudes and new-found skills around audit and feedback to embed the innovation. They were helped in this by a series of organisation-wide actions that were orchestrated by the expert team of facilitators in collaboration with the senior executive team (which included the Chief Executive Officer, Director of Nursing, Heads of Dietetics and Catering Services). The expert facilitators ensured that appropriate attention was given to the provision of ongoing education and support for all staff on this topic; that relevant changes were made to the existing policies and procedures to incorporate the changes; that communication about the project was sent out to all relevant stakeholders and that a process improvement plan was actioned around areas of service delivery (e.g. management of stores and requisitions, purchase of equipment such as refrigerators and weighing machines) which was vital to ensure the longer term sustainability of the improvements.

The final part of the experienced facilitator's armoury around capacity development and sustainability is well summarised in the work of Bate et al. (2008). They identified six dimensions that are important in sustaining achievements in quality within organisations through a series of case studies in healthcare organisations with a reputation for leading improvement. These were described as structural, political, cultural, educational, emotional and physical/technological factors. As outlined in Table 7.3, these dimensions reflect the underlying skill

TABLE 7.3 Core dimensions of organising for quality and operationalisation through the facilitator's role

Dimension	Activity as demonstrated through the facilitator role
Structural	Planning and coordinating Making sure you get the right structures in place
Political	Negotiating change and managing conflict Recognising and dealing with conflicts and tensions that emerge early on
Cultural	Giving the activity (introducing a new piece of evidence or innovation or improvement) a shared, collective meaning Building a sense of cohesion and strong team effort
Educational	Learning through doing and reflecting on this Learning by your mistakes and using them to improve
Emotional	Motivating Feeling and sharing the highs and lows of working together on a project and as a team
Physical/technological	Understanding the design of technical and other systems Not putting all your trust in technological or systems solutions – they are only as good as the people using them!

Source: After Bate et al. (2008).

set of the facilitator – being able to plan (structure), negotiate and manage conflict (political), building a sense of cohesion and teamwork (cultural), enabling learning on the job and through experience (education), motivating others (emotional) and knowing how to get the best from the physical resources in the system (physical/technological).

Masso et al. (2014) drew upon Normalisation Process Theory and the 'Organising for Quality' framework developed by Bate et al. (2008) as a way of explaining how a number of innovations were introduced into aged care facilities across Australia. They found that it was the ability of teams to understand and share experiences that led them 'to make sense' of the new innovation in their daily routines and determined the uptake and eventual adoption and sustaining of the change. This overarching construct was termed 'on common ground' (Masso et al., 2014) and embedded within this were experiences of learning by connecting, the ability to reconcile competing priorities and feeling in control or able to exercise agency. A key finding was that facilitation was variable across the sites, leading the research team to speculate whether the adoption process could have been improved if the facilitators had been more coordinated.

These sources of theoretical and empirical evidence reinforce the view that the adoption, embedding and sustaining of any innovation is a social process involving learning and behaviour change as well as changes in the structure (policies, procedures, work practices) of the organisation. Aligning all of these facets is part of the work of the experienced and expert facilitator.

The expert facilitator: capacity development, mentoring, sustaining and spreading change

The expert facilitator role is one of coordination, leadership and the provision of high-level expertise around the four dimensions of the i-PARIHS framework. The expert facilitator may be located within one organisation, but more commonly they work across organisations and in particular bridge the academic–healthcare organisation boundary. In recent years there has been much interest in the formalisation of such facilitation networks, in particular within primary care. The Agency for Healthcare Research and Quality published a facilitation guide that outlines how practice facilitation networks can be established with the primary objective of improving the uptake and adoption of new evidence into primary care practice (Knox et al., 2011). Networks in the United States, Canada and Australia have been using this approach (Nagykaldi et al., 2005; Knox et al., 2011; Liddy et al., 2013). It is within the role and remit of experienced and expert facilitators to establish networks such as these. There is also a growing body of evidence of the effectiveness of these practice facilitation approaches, not just in terms of evidence of impact (Baskerville et al., 2012), but also in terms of the longer term sustainability of the change by using facilitation as the primary intervention (Hogg et al., 2008).

The example of the management of chronic kidney disease in primary care in the UK (see Chapter 8) also illustrates the partnership working between academic and service areas with expert facilitators and researchers identifying and supporting novice facilitators to introduce improvements within a primary care setting.

The expert facilitation role therefore needs to be positioned at a strategic level with the authority to influence behaviours and actions across multiple systems. In this sense, they would be expert in understanding and dealing with the outer system level contextual challenges as identified in the i-PARIHS framework: engaging stakeholders; understanding the politics and power relations; knowing how to communicate the initiative in clear, concise terms and being able to move between and across multiple boundaries. In addition to these political negotiating skills, the expert facilitator would have a set of technical and process skills that built on the theoretical underpinnings and practices of the i-PARIHS framework, as well as additional skills and capabilities in evaluation and research.

Many expert facilitators will find themselves being part of large-scale implementation research programmes where they will be responsible for ensuring the introduction of the facilitation intervention. This requires a deep understanding of what elements of the intervention can be standardised and how local adaptation and refinement needs to be acknowledged as part of the implementation process and the facilitator's skill in interpreting contextual variation.

The expert facilitator will be responsible for guiding and supporting a network of experienced or local facilitators within a larger scale initiative. They need to consider how they provide mentorship and support and how they keep the local facilitators on track (Nagykaldi et al., 2005). The case studies reported in Chapters 9, 10 and 12 describe a range of challenges for expert facilitators working across cultural and language barriers (Chapters 9 and 10), challenges of providing virtual support across time zones (Chapters 9 and 12) and countries and the challenge of not being able to select local facilitators for the programme (Chapter 9).

The expert facilitator role takes responsibility for the integrity of the facilitation process and thereby is in a position to begin to explore it in a more systematic and structured way. By outlining the practical steps and framing these within a theoretical framework, it is possible to begin to test out different aspects of the overall implementation process. The expert facilitator may find themselves as part of a larger research team that is looking at these issues. This may involve using a range of different research methods, from in-depth qualitative case studies to randomised controlled trials, as the case studies in this book illustrate. Given the complexities of implementation, it is particularly useful to think about research and evaluation designs that help to uncover and understand what is happening, for example, at the level of the innovation, the recipients and the inner and outer context. This may mean undertaking a process evaluation alongside a more conventional trial, adopting a theory-driven approach such as realist evaluation, or using a participatory action research design. Building an understanding of these different methodologies and how they can add to the science of implementation is an important area in which the expert facilitator can contribute to bridging the worlds of practice, research and theory. Box 7.1 provides some suggestions for further reading around researching implementation.

BOX 7.1 SUGGESTIONS FOR FURTHER READING AROUND RESEARCHING IMPLEMENTATION

Books

Ovretveit, J. 2002. *Action Evaluation of Health Programmes and Changes – A Handbook for a User-focused Approach*. Oxford: Radcliffe.
Ovretveit, J. 2014. *Evaluating Improvement and Evaluation for Health*. Maidenhead, Berkshire: Open University Press.
Pawson, R. 2013. *The Science of Evaluation: A Realist Manifesto*. London: Sage.
Pawson, R. & Tilley, N. 1997. *Realistic Evaluation*. Thousand Oaks, CA: Sage.

(continued)

(continued)

Journal

Implementation Science is an online journal that specifically aims to 'publish research relevant to the scientific study of methods to promote the uptake of research findings into routine healthcare in clinical, organisational or policy contexts' www.implementationscience.com/

The expert facilitator role spans the worlds of practice and research. It can be located in academia with strong links to practice or it can be based in a healthcare organisation with links to an academic institution. What is most important is the continual connection of these two worldviews. The growing development of Academic Health Science Centres and Networks in countries such as the United Kingdom and Australia confirms this recognition that knowledge translation – or the movement of evidence into practice – is as much an interactive and dynamic process as it is about the instrumental movement of knowledge products from one group of people to another. The expert facilitator role needs to understand the complexities involved, at the same time as having the practical know-how to enable individuals, teams and units to work effectively together. Applying learning from contemporary research into networks and communities of practice (Le May, 2009; Ferlie et al., 2013; Rycroft-Malone et al., 2013) should help to develop more advanced understanding around the sorts of processes and structures that need to be established to enable this type of learning and spread of knowledge.

Some final thoughts on capacity development, sustainability and spread

We are still in a period of development and exploration in terms of formalising the role of the facilitator and understanding how that influences and impacts on the wider system. There have been some important developments in models such as primary care facilitation (Knox et al., 2011) and the growth of academic–health service partnerships to engage in the development and implementation of applied research to improve patient care and population health (for example, see the case study reported in Chapter 8 describing a Collaboration for Applied Health Research and Care (CLAHRC) in the English National Health Service).

There is also growing recognition that the worlds of quality improvement, knowledge translation and evidence-based practice need to work more closely together (Harvey, 2005). The methods at the heart of the Facilitator's Toolkit are central to healthcare improvement methodology. Research consistently affirms the importance of audit and feedback on performance as one way to help individuals reflect upon their practice and think about ways to improve (Jamtvedt et al., 2006; Ivers et al., 2012). Equally, the evidence around the need to embed innovations into routines is growing – the notion which Lewin (1947) identified as unfreezing, changing and (re)freezing would seem to be a profound requirement in any system to ensure that innovations are embraced and sustained. Yet at the same time, the organisation needs to remain vigilant and open to new knowledge and further innovation. The final question is how do we speed up the spread of innovations? Again we seem to be moving towards a position where spread is viewed as a deeply social phenomenon – it is about networks of individuals talking and sharing, discovering and feeling a sense of connectivity, excitement, exploration and – as Masso et al. (2014) described, being on 'common ground'. That shared understanding (of the problem or challenge), the desire to experiment and improve and the determination to change one's routines and habits in the light of that experience are at the core of capacity development, sustainability and spread (Bate et al., 2004). There is more to discover about how to develop, foster and learn from social networks and communities of practice within healthcare settings.

In the facilitation model we have proposed, we are suggesting that the roles of experienced and expert facilitators contribute to this important agenda. However, we also acknowledge that the evidence to substantiate this claim is emergent and in need of further development and refinement. Our aim in writing this chapter has been to lay out the arguments; this represents a basis from which future research can be undertaken in order to test the related assumptions and propositions. We will return to this in the final chapter.

References

Baskerville, N.B., Liddy, C. & Hogg, W. 2012. Systematic review and meta-analysis of practice facilitation within primary care settings. *Annals of Family Medicine*, 10, 63–74.

Bate, P., Robert, G. & Bevan, H. 2004. The next phase of healthcare improvement: what can we learn from social movements? *Quality and Safety in Health Care*, 13, 62–6.

Bate, P., Mendel, P. & Robert, G. 2008. *Organising for Quality: The Improvement Journeys of Leading Hospitals in Europe and the United States*. Abingdon: Radcliffe.

Ferlie, E., McGivern, G. & Fitzgerald, L. 2013. *Making Wicked Problems Governable? The Case of Managed Networks in Health Care*. Oxford: Oxford University Press.

Gordge, L., De Young, J. & Wiechula, R. 2009. Reducing functional decline of older people in an acute-care setting: are we providing adequate care to maintain/optimise the functional status of our elder patients? *International Journal of Evidence Based Healthcare*, 7, 181–6.

Harvey, G. 2005. Quality improvement and evidence-based practice: as one or at odds in the effort to promote better health care? *Worldviews on Evidence-Based Nursing*, 2, 52–4.

Hogg, W., Lemelin, J., Moroz, I., Soto, E. & Russell, G. 2008. Improving prevention in primary care: Evaluating the sustainability of outreach facilitation. *Canadian Family Physician*, 54, 712–20.

Ivers, N., Jamtvedt, G., Flottorp, S., Young, J.M., Odgaard-Jensen, J., French, S.D., O'Brien, M.A., Johansen, M., Grimshaw, J. & Oxman, A.D. 2012. Audit and feedback: effects on professional practice and healthcare outcomes. *Cochrane Database of Systematic Reviews*, 6, CD000259.

Jamtvedt, G., Young, J.M., Kristoffersen, D.T., O'Brien, M.A. & Oxman, A.D. 2006. Does telling people what they have been doing change what they do? A systematic review of the effects of audit and feedback. *Quality and Safety in Health Care*, 15, 433–6.

Kislov, R., Waterman, H., Harvey, G. & Boaden, R. 2014. Rethinking capacity building for knowledge mobilisation: developing multilevel capabilities in healthcare organisations. *Implementation Science*, 9, 166.

Kitson, A., Wiechula, R., Zeitz, K., Marcionni, D., Page, T. & Silverston, H. 2011. Improving older peoples' care in one acute hospital setting: a realist evaluation of a KT intervention. Adelaide: University of Adelaide.

Kitson, A., Marcionni, D., Page, T., Wiechula, R., Zeitz, K. & Silverston, H. 2010. Using knowledge translation to transform the fundamentals of care: the older person and improving care project. In: Lyons, R. F. (ed.) *Using Evidence: Advances and Debates in Bridging Health Research and Action*. Halifax, Canada: Atlantic Health Promotion Research Centre, Dalhousie University.

Knox, L., Taylor, E., Geonnotti, K., Machta, R., Kim, J., Nysenbaum, J. & Parchman, M. 2011. *Developing and Running a Primary Care Practice Facilitation Program: A How-to Guide*. Rockville, MD: Agency for Healthcare Research and Quality.

Le May, A. 2009. *Communities of Practice in Health and Social Care.* Oxford: Wiley-Blackwell.

Lewin, K. 1947. Frontiers in group dynamics. In: Cartwright, D. (ed.) *Field Theory in Social Science.* London: Social Science Paperbacks.

Liddy, C., Laferriere, D., Baskerville, B., Dahrouge, S., Knox, L. & Hogg, W. 2013. An overview of practice facilitation programs in Canada: current perspectives and future directions. *Healthcare Policy*, 8, 58–67.

Masso, M., McCarthy, G. & Kitson, A. 2014. Mechanisms which help explain implementation of evidence-based practice in residential aged care facilities: a grounded theory study. *International Journal of Nursing Studies*, 51, 1014–26.

May, C. & Finch, T. 2009. Implementation, embedding, and integration: an outline of Normalization Process Theory. *Sociology*, 43, 535–54.

McLiesh, P., Mungall, D. & Wiechula, R. 2009. Are we providing the best possible pain management for our elderly patients in the acute-care setting? *International Journal of Evidence-Based Healthcare*, 7, 173–80.

Nagykaldi, Z., Mold, J.W. & Aspy, C.B. 2005. Practice facilitators: a review of the literature. *Family Medicine*, 37, 581–8.

Rycroft-Malone, J., Wilkinson, J., Burton, C.R., Harvey, G., McCormack, B., Graham, I. & Staniszewska, S. 2013. Collaborative action around implementation in Collaborations for Leadership in Applied Health Research and Care: towards a programme theory. *Journal of Health Services Research & Policy*, 18, 13–26.

Wiechula, R., Kitson, A., Marcoionni, D., Page, T., Zeitz, K. & Silverston, H. 2009. Improving the fundamentals of care for older people in the acute hospital setting: facilitating practice improvement using a Knowledge Translation Toolkit. *International Journal of Evidence-Based Healthcare*, 7, 283–95.

8

FACILITATION METHODS WITHIN A PROJECT TO IMPROVE THE MANAGEMENT OF CHRONIC KIDNEY DISEASE IN PRIMARY CARE

Gill Harvey, Janet Hegarty, John Humphreys, Katy Rothwell, Roman Kislov, Viv Entwistle and Ruth Boaden

Introduction and background to the facilitation project

This case study presents a project undertaken in the English National Health Service (NHS) to improve the identification and management of chronic kidney disease (CKD) in primary care, using a range of facilitation strategies. These included specially appointed facilitator roles working in a wider facilitation team, the use of structured improvement methods and processes, stakeholder engagement, collaborative learning and networking. We begin the chapter by outlining the background to the project, including how the focus for implementation activities was identified. We then describe how we developed our approach to facilitating implementation, describing both the facilitator roles and the facilitation strategies that were employed by the implementation team to identify and address agreed goals, engage with key stakeholders and assess and manage the contextual issues. Evaluation data relating to the processes and outcomes of implementation will be presented before we conclude the chapter by reflecting on the practical lessons we have learnt about facilitation – our 'top ten' tips for how to successfully facilitate an implementation project. We will finally summarise what we believe our experiences add to the knowledge base about facilitating evidence-based healthcare.

The focus on chronic kidney disease

The project we are describing was undertaken within a large initiative aimed at translating research evidence into practice. In 2008, in response to national concerns about the recognised gaps between the production of research and its uptake in routine healthcare, nine Collaborations for Leadership in Applied Health Research and Care (CLAHRCs) were established as partnerships between higher education and local NHS organisations. One of the nine CLAHRCs was in Greater Manchester (CLAHRC GM), a collaboration between the University of Manchester and 19 local NHS partners (10 primary care, 5 acute, 3 mental health, 1 ambulance). The CLAHRC received a total of £20 million in funding over a 5-year period from 2008 to 2013; £10 million of funding came from the National Institute for Health Research and a further £10 million of matched funding was provided by local primary care organisations (known as primary care trusts). [Note: At the start of the CLAHRC, these organisations were called primary care trusts or PCTs and functioned as a mostly administrative body, responsible for commissioning primary, community and secondary health services from providers. As such, PCTs were responsible for spending around 80% of the total NHS budget. PCTs were abolished on 31 March 2013, to be replaced by clinical commissioning groups (CCGs).] The focus of CLAHRC GM was on improving cardiovascular health in the population of Greater Manchester and as part of this strategy one of the disease areas selected was CKD, which is known to be a key influence on the risk of cardiovascular disease (Go et al., 2004).

Knowledge and awareness of CKD has grown since the publication of an international classification system in 2002 (K/DOQI, 2002). This classification grades CKD from stages 1 to 5, with stage 5 representing end-stage kidney disease, with the associated high cost of management and treatment via dialysis and/or transplantation. CKD is now recognised as a significant public health issue, with an estimated worldwide prevalence between 8 and 16%, which increases greatly with age. It is relatively 'silent' in the earlier stages; however, if the condition is not managed (for example, through reduction of blood pressure), the chances of an individual with CKD suffering a cardiovascular event such as stroke are significantly increased. Furthermore, without management, the likelihood of progressing to more advanced CKD is greater. The key to management is slowing down the progression of the disease, through regular monitoring and interventions to control blood pressure and proteinuria (the presence of excess serum proteins in the urine, which, in patients with kidney disease, is indicative of an insufficiency of protein absorption or impaired filtration), including modifications to lifestyle and diet. Before such planned interventions become possible, there is a need to accurately identify and assess individuals in the population with CKD.

At the start of the project, national statistics suggested the prevalence of CKD in the UK adult population to be 8.5% (Stevens et al., 2007). We used existing national and local general practice data to assess the current level of CKD care provision in primary care (Health and Social Care Information Centre, http://qof.hscic.gov.uk/index.asp). In 2008/9, the recorded prevalence of CKD in Greater Manchester was 4.1%, significantly lower than national estimates. The same data also indicated that of those patients on existing registers, approximately 30% were not receiving optimal disease management, such as monitoring of their blood pressure or testing for proteinuria. This was the starting point for the project – an attempt to implement available evidence for the identification and management of CKD in a primary care setting.

The evidence base for identifying and managing CKD in primary care

UK national clinical guidelines on the identification and management of adults with CKD in primary care were published around the same time as the project commenced (NICE, 2008). Similar clinical guidelines also exist at an international level, reinforcing the importance of identifying people in the population with early-stage CKD and actively managing the condition to reduce potential longer term effects (K/DOQI, 2002). However, the existence of evidence summaries such as clinical guidelines is rarely sufficient to change practice, as the growing evidence base on the uptake and implementation of guidelines demonstrates (Grimshaw et al., 2004). The challenge therefore was to develop an implementation strategy that recognised the existence of the guidelines, but sought to actively facilitate their implementation within general practice in Greater Manchester.

Overview of the facilitation approach

Because the CKD project was part of the wider CLAHRC initiative, there were a number of parallel projects taking place that focused on different issues relating to cardiovascular health, for example, stroke and diabetes. Collectively, we worked together to agree an implementation framework for the CLAHRC programme of work. This framework was developed by reviewing the available theoretical and empirical literature on implementing evidence-based healthcare, alongside our own personal experiences of the processes – and challenges – involved in implementation (Harvey et al., 2011). This resulted in a framework that comprised four key elements:

- the PARIHS (Promoting Action on Research Implementation in Health Services) framework with its core elements of evidence, context and facilitation framing the implementation process (Kitson et al., 1998; Rycroft-Malone et al., 2002);
- a modified version of the Model for Improvement (Langley et al., 1996) which through its three key components (What are we trying to accomplish? How will we know that a change is an improvement? What changes can we make that will result in improvement?) provided a way to operationalise implementation;
- multi-professional teams to facilitate implementation, including individuals in designated facilitator roles; and
- embedded evaluation and learning to ensure real-time evaluation and modification to projects as required.

Elements of the CKD facilitation strategy

Using these four elements, we designed the CKD project and facilitation strategy.

The PARIHS framework provided the initial points of reference for the facilitation strategy, highlighting that successful implementation was going to depend on successfully translating – via our facilitation approach – the evidence about CKD within the local context, which comprised multiple general practices in different regions of Greater Manchester.

Building on the Model for Improvement, we set the project up along the lines of an improvement collaborative (IHI, 2003). This applies the principles of the Model for Improvement within a 12-month structured programme for multiple participating organisations or teams, encompassing joint learning events, agreed goals for improvement, action periods using Plan–Do–Study–Act (PDSA) cycles, regular data collection and feedback and ongoing project support. The two collaboratives described in the chapter took place between September 2009 and March 2012.

The third element of the strategy was a multi-professional team to design and facilitate the collaborative. In this case, the team was made up of: a part-time clinical lead who was a kidney consultant with expert knowledge about the condition; a part-time academic lead with knowledge and experience in facilitating implementation; a programme manager; an information analyst; and two newly appointed facilitators (with the title of knowledge transfer associates, KTAs) to act as the key points of contact between general practices and the project team. The facilitators were recruited at the start of the CLAHRC. They did not have prior NHS experience, but were recruited on the basis of their problem-solving and interpersonal skills following a two-day assessment panel. This meant that the facilitators started as novices in the role, both in terms of the context in which they working (a general practice setting within the NHS) and the requirements of the role, namely to facilitate the translation of research evidence into general practice.

The final element of the facilitation approach was formative evaluation and learning, which as well as being part of the implementation research strategy, provided an important source of development and support for the novice facilitators. This was primarily achieved through monthly meetings of the project team to analyse the progress of participating general practices and provide mentorship and support to the facilitators, as will be described more fully later in the chapter. In addition to this project level evaluation, the facilitators participated in a cooperative inquiry group, which was established for all the KTAs appointed to the CLAHRC, to provide a mechanism for reflective learning, development and support in the role. (Note: Derived from ideas of participatory action research, a cooperative inquiry group involves individuals with similar interests and concerns working collectively to share, reflect and learn from their experiences.) Monthly learning and support sessions for the KTAs conducted for the first two years of the CLAHRC provided another source of education and development for the facilitator role, covering topics such as group dynamics, context assessment, negotiation and presentation skills.

To summarise, the key point to highlight in terms of the facilitation approach we adopted is that we had a designated team to support implementation, bringing a range of knowledge, skills and routes of influence to the project. This team included individuals in designated practice facilitator roles, as part of a multi-faceted intervention that was based upon the design of an improvement collaborative. This approach supported the sharing of ideas between practices, as well as two-way learning between the facilitators and the organisations they were working with. However, we were particularly cognisant of the need to be responsive to contextual issues at the local level and built in ways to tailor the facilitation approach at an individual practice level; this will be illustrated further as we move though the chapter.

Implementing the evidence: project design

As indicated, the starting point for the project was awareness that the recorded prevalence of CKD was lower than would be expected. This suggested that there were large numbers of people with undiagnosed CKD in the population of Greater Manchester and within both the diagnosed and undiagnosed population there was recognised poor care of patients with CKD. Clinical guidelines had recently been produced (NICE, 2008) providing an up-to-date summary of the evidence on how to identify and manage CKD in primary care. One of the first steps was to convene an expert stakeholder group to agree the aims for the collaborative and a framework for change (commonly known as a driver diagram) (Figure 8.1). This group included patient representatives, primary and secondary care experts, improvement specialists and local stakeholders and met prior to the start of the first improvement collaborative.

The first collaborative involved 19 general practices located within four different primary care trusts (PCTs); the second involved 11 practices, mostly drawn from one PCT. In both cases, practices were requested to identify a small multi-professional improvement team, ideally comprising representation from the medical, nursing and administrative members of the practice. This team participated in three collaborative learning events. The learning events took place at the start of the collaborative, then at around four months and eight months with a

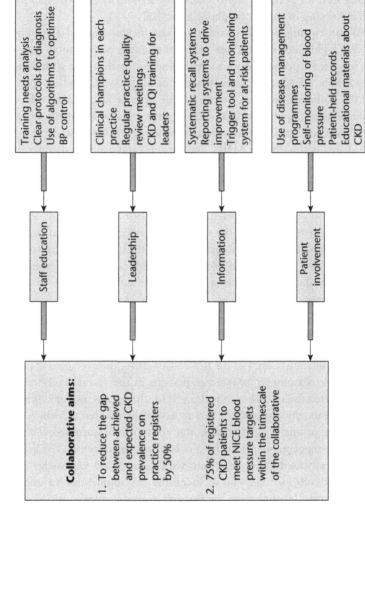

FIGURE 8.1 The CLAHRC GM CKD collaborative driver diagram

final closing/celebratory meeting at the end of the collaborative. The learning events included some formal presentations, for example, on the condition of CKD and evidence about how best to manage it and on working effectively in teams, alongside opportunities for informal networking and information sharing among participants. In between the learning events, the practice improvement teams were expected to work with their colleagues in the wider practice to introduce small tests of change using PDSA cycles. Each practice was supported by one of the facilitators who visited regularly to discuss progress and offer support, for example, by suggesting areas for potential improvement and sharing ideas from other participating practices, as well as keeping in contact by phone and email.

All participating practices worked towards the same agreed goals (Figure 8.1) and the driver diagram highlighted the key areas where they might want to focus their action cycles, although this was left for practice teams to determine during meetings with their facilitator. Prevalence targets were calculated for each practice individually, depending upon their starting position and the estimated prevalence value for the practice (according to the demographic make-up of the practice population). All practices were required to submit monthly data relating to the prevalence and blood pressure management goals. These data were collated by the information analyst within the CLAHRC project team and practices then received monthly feedback, illustrating their own progress and how this compared to the averages for the collaborative as a whole in the style of a dashboard report (Figure 8.2).

One final element of the implementation approach was the provision of financial reimbursement to participating practices. Most GPs in the NHS are self-employed, therefore, a provision was made within the CLAHRC budget to 'buy out' time for the improvement teams to attend learning events and undertake the implementation work back in their practice. Although these payments did not cover the full cost of involvement, they were intended to make a contribution to covering time for key staff to be involved. In the first collaborative, additional staged payments were made to practices when they reached key milestones, such as attendance at the learning events and achievement of improvement targets. Although a detailed economic analysis was not undertaken, it was possible to estimate the cost of running the project, in terms of the practice payments and the costs associated with the collaborative and the facilitation team. For the first collaborative, the average cost per practice was £20,000; this halved to around £10,000 per practice in the second collaborative. This reduction in costs occurred for a number of reasons. First, the money available from the CLAHRC for the second collaborative was lower due to economic constraints, which resulted in less financial support for practices and fewer/shorter collaborative learning events (half a day rather than a full day), supplemented by virtual online seminars. Second, the learning from the first collaborative provided the project team with an increased knowledge base from which to start the second collaborative. This included the development of an improvement guide, which summarised the learning from the first collaborative and was provided to practices starting out on the second collaborative. Third, at the time of the first collaborative, a research team in another CLAHRC had developed a software programme that could identify and check CKD patients on practice registers (IMPAKT™, 2013). This audit software was made available for the practices participating in the second collaborative and effectively reduced the amount of time and support that was needed to identify patients with CKD.

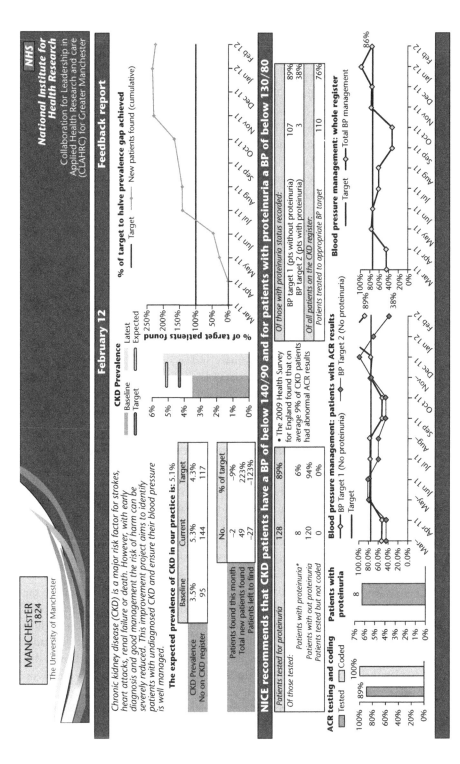

FIGURE 8.2 Example of a practice dashboard report

Methods used to identify and work with stakeholders

The importance of stakeholder engagement was recognised from the outset of the project, particularly given the number of organisations participating and the fact that the PCTs were contributing financially to the work of the CLAHRC. Once the four PCTs to be involved in the first collaborative had been agreed, an initial process of stakeholder mapping was undertaken to identify key individuals who could influence and, in turn, needed to be involved and kept informed about the programme of work on CKD. These included chief executives and senior managers in the four PCTs, GPs with a leadership role, public health specialists and commissioners of specialist services. Meetings were arranged with these individuals to explain the purpose and aims of the project; these meetings typically involved the senior leaders of the CLAHRC, along with the programme manager and clinical lead. One outcome was the identification of a senior sponsor in each PCT to act as a key point of contact with the CKD project team. The senior sponsors received regular updates on the progress of the project within the practices that reported to their organisation and were also approached on an 'as needs' basis if particular issues or barriers to implementation were identified.

The expert stakeholder group meeting represented another form of stakeholder engagement, ensuring that a wider group of patient, clinical and academic experts had an opportunity to agree on the evidence and input to the implementation strategy. This group also received regular feedback on the progress of the project and members of the expert faculty were invited to participate in the learning events to discuss issues of CKD from different perspectives, such as the patient perspective, or the secondary care view. Interactions such as these helped to provide an important link between primary and secondary care relating to the management of patients with CKD. Finally, at an overall level the collaborative was chaired by a kidney consultant who was the lead for renal disease at a national level in the NHS, providing an important communication channel between the project and national level policy.

Methods used to assess and respond to contextual issues

Although the collaborative methodology provides a relatively structured framework for implementation, the importance of being responsive to local contextual issues was central to the design of the project. This required the identification of ways to incorporate local context assessment and tailoring of interventions into the overall design and conduct of the project, which was achieved through a number of different means. Informed by the PARIHS sub-elements of context (McCormack et al., 2002), we undertook an initial short baseline survey in participating practices to assess elements of culture, leadership and orientation towards learning and evaluation. All staff within the practice were encouraged to complete the survey and results were then collated and fed back to the practice by the facilitators to discuss the findings and, in particular, factors that were likely to enable or inhibit the process of implementation (for example, the extent to which staff felt involved in decision-making, the leadership style of senior managers, familiarity with clinical guidelines and audit). The facilitators then used these data to plan their visits to individual practices and identify specific topics for discussion, such as how best to engage the whole practice team in the project.

The fact that facilitators were visiting the practices in person also gave them the opportunity to build relationships with practice staff and develop a better understanding of the local context. This in turn helped to interpret the monthly data on practice progress against the two main aims. The CLAHRC facilitation team met monthly to review progress against the key targets. This was tracked using run charts with data plotted for individual practices and for the collaborative as a whole. Where points of variance were identified, a more in-depth analysis of what was happening in the practice took place, informed by the facilitator's observations and insights from their interaction with the practice. One framework that was helpful in this respect was that developed by Bate and colleagues from their analysis of organisations that had successfully implemented and sustained quality improvement in healthcare (Bate et al., 2008). This framework identifies six key areas – described as core challenges – that can influence the organisational improvement trajectory, namely, structural, political, cultural, educational, emotional and physical/technological challenges. Table 8.1 outlines how and why these six factors are seen to exert an influence on the implementation and improvement journey. The framework complemented the context dimension of the PARIHS framework and provided a useful way to structure a discussion around practice progress in order to identify what facilitator interventions might be appropriate. Table 8.2 provides a summary of a practice review using this approach.

In some cases, issues were identified that were particularly problematic to address, for example, a senior GP who refused to accept CKD as a disease and was proving difficult to get on board in terms of supporting the changes that were needed or improvement teams who appeared to be dysfunctional in the ways they were working. During the review process, ideas were put forward about how best to handle the issues that were presenting during implementation and which members of the project team needed to be involved in addressing them. For some issues, this was simply a case of agreeing strategies that the facilitators could use in their next practice visit; however, in other cases, the plan involved other members of the project team working alongside the facilitators to provide additional mentorship and support. This was particularly so when the barriers faced were more difficult. For example, in the case of a senior GP being unsupportive or actively opposing the proposed changes, the strategy involved the clinical lead in the project paying the practice a visit in order to use their clinical influence with medical colleagues. Another parallel action may have been to arrange a meeting with the senior sponsor for the project to discuss the issues and seek their support. However, these plans were made on a case-by-case basis depending on the nature of the problem, the stage of the project and the facilitator's detailed knowledge of the practice and the staff involved.

At the end of the first collaborative, one of the practice nurses who had been a member of an improvement team was seconded to work part-time as a facilitator within the second collaborative. This was a deliberate strategy to develop implementation capability at a local level,

TABLE 8.1 Six core challenges in organising for quality

Area of challenge	Concerned with . . .	What happens if neglected
Structural	Planning and coordination	Fragmentation
Political	Negotiating change and managing conflict	Disillusionment and inertia
Cultural	Giving quality a shared, collective meaning	Evaporation
Educational	Learning and accumulating knowledge	Amnesia and frustration
Emotional	Motivating	Loss of interest
Physical/technological	Design of technical and other systems	Exhaustion

Source: After Bate et al. (2008).

TABLE 8.2 Example of a project team practice review discussion

Area of challenge	Assessment	Comment/follow-up actions
Structural	Lack of synergy with other staff, lack of synergy within QI team could be a problem	Noticeable in the staff room; even though they are on their break, the staff have no awareness or interest in the project. Are they ready to tackle this? Need to work with improvement team to find ways to generate greater staff engagement
Political	No obvious issues, although the practice manager is newly appointed; is negotiating change with the other staff an issue?	Discuss with the improvement team when considering ways to bring other staff on board
Cultural	There is little embedded QI in the practice and the changes could evaporate after the collaborative if there is no spread to the other staff	Bring other staff in more – involve them in smaller tests of change? Bring them in on other disease areas?
Educational	Lack of awareness of the skills they are developing; risk that change will not be sustained	Need to use PDSA worksheets more to make them think about the work they are doing and therefore embed the skills a bit more
Emotional	Loss of motivation is a risk due to the perception that there is no real change	Need to show graph of number of patients tested for proteinuria, number of additional patients found and highlight impact of that on patient care (number of strokes prevented etc.)
Physical/ technological	Lack of time to make changes may be an issue and the computer does not always return accurate search results	Work with the practice staff to create accurate searches; encourage them to take up some locum cover to free up their time

Abbreviation: QI, quality improvement; PDSA, Plan–Do–Study–Act.

in anticipation of the time when the CLAHRC projects ended. This new facilitator was somewhat different from the KTA facilitators. She had insider knowledge, in terms of the practice setting (the practices in the second collaborative were mostly from the same geographical area where the practice nurse worked), of the local politics that existed and of the change processes involved in implementation. This was particularly beneficial to the project in terms of identifying, understanding and managing contextual issues at a local level as the facilitator had clinical credibility and a range of personal knowledge and experience to draw on when working with colleagues to facilitate and support implementation. In addition, the facilitator had a formal and informal network of contacts within the local geographical area which helped in terms of anticipating and troubleshooting problems.

Evaluating the impact of facilitation

Improvements were noted in both the identification of patients with CKD and management of their condition according to evidence-based guidelines. Overall, the recorded prevalence of CKD increased by 1.2%, suggesting improvements at a practice level in case finding and equating to an additional 1863 patients added to practice CKD registers. In relation to the second improvement target, management of blood pressure (BP) in line with national guidelines also improved; 74% and 83% (1st and 2nd collaborative, respectively) of patients on practice registers had BP maintained within the NICE specified guideline recommendations by the end of the 12-month period. Table 8.3 summarises the main findings in relation to the collaborative goals.

Although these data indicate improvements in the identification and management of CKD, it is important to note the limitations of a 'before and after' measure such as this. Using the national pay for performance data (Health and Social Care Information Centre), we were able to make some comparisons between the practices involved in the improvement collaborative and practices that were not involved. Although a general trend of improvement in the care of patients with CKD is apparent (perhaps unsurprisingly as general practices were receiving financial incentives to address this aspect of care via the national primary care pay for performance system), the level of improvement in the collaborative practices appeared to be greater. For example, over the same time period as the collaborative project, the increase in nationally recorded prevalence rates of CKD was no greater than 0.2%, compared to a 1.2% improvement in participating practices. Similar findings were apparent with comparisons around the BP target, where comparisons within one geographical region indicated that achievement of the BP target was around 8% higher over a 12-month period in the participating practices. However, we recognise that in order to rigorously evaluate the impact of the intervention (i.e. improvement collaborative with tailored facilitation), a controlled study with matched intervention and non-intervention sites would be required.

TABLE 8.3 Summary of achievement of collaborative goals

Collaborative goal	Practices in first collaborative (n = 19)		Practices in second collaborative (n = 11)	
	Average baseline prevalence across practices at the start of the collaborative	Average prevalence after 12 months	Average baseline prevalence across practices at the start of the collaborative	Average prevalence after 12 months
To reduce the gap between achieved and expected CKD prevalence on practice registers by 50%	3.9% prevalence	5.1% prevalence	4.6% prevalence	5.8% prevalence
75% of registered CKD patients to meet NICE BP targets within the timescale of the collaborative	34% of patients diagnosed with CKD managed according to BP targets	74% of patients diagnosed with CKD managed according to BP targets	58% of patients diagnosed with CKD managed according to BP targets	83% of patients diagnosed with CKD managed according to BP targets

Abbreviations: CKD, chronic kidney disease; NICE, National Institute for Health and Care Excellence; BP, blood pressure.

Analysis of the process data collected during the course of working with the practices revealed a number of enabling factors that were common across the sites. Features of the collaborative approach – notably the joint learning events, the establishment of clear aims and regular feedback of data – generally acted as enablers of improvement, as did the ongoing support from facilitators and the provision of financial reimbursement. A particular barrier in the first collaborative was the lack of knowledge and skills at practice level to extract the required data, compounded by the multiple different record systems that were used in primary care. This barrier was much less of an issue in the second collaborative when the IMPAKT™ audit software programme was included as part of the implementation strategy.

Considerable variation was apparent in terms of the progress made at an individual practice level, despite the observed improvement at an overall level. For example, in the first collaborative, only 10 of the 19 practices achieved the prevalence target and 9 achieved the BP target (Humphreys et al., 2012). In the second collaborative, the figures were 7 out of 11 and 11 out of 11, respectively. This suggests a more consistent level of achievement in phase 2, yet still a level of variation exists. The process evaluation identified a number of factors accounting for the different levels of progress that individual practices made. These included how important the topic of CKD was for the practice, how much support was provided by the senior leadership, how receptive the practice culture was to change and how involved the whole practice team were in the improvement project (Rothwell et al., 2012). These observations reflect similar findings from other studies of improvement collaboratives in healthcare (for example, Øvretveit et al., 2002).

Reflections and lessons learnt

In order to reflect on our experiences and the lessons learnt during the first few years of facilitating the improvement of CKD in primary care, individual members of the project team each listed the top five things they felt they had learnt about facilitation. We then analysed and themed the responses to identify our top ten lessons about facilitation from this particular project. These are as follows – starting with the issues that were mentioned most frequently amongst the team – and illustrated with some representative quotes to reflect the points identified.

Lesson 1: Make the work manageable: 'chunk it down'

All members of the team identified this as a priority, in order to make the aims seem achievable from both the facilitator's perspective and the staff involved in the project at a practice level. This is reflected in the following quotes:

> Participating in a project with ambitious aims can initially feel very overwhelming for all involved, particularly in the context of healthcare improvement projects where staff view the project as something they are doing 'in addition to their day-to-day job'. A valuable and key role of a facilitator is to break the project down into manageable pieces, or 'bitesize chunks' – separate sets of tasks which they gradually introduce to participants over time. This enables staff to focus on achieving manageable short-term or 'mini-goals', which, over time, collectively enable them to achieve the overall aim. (KTA 2)
>
> Try not to overload an already busy member of staff, approach with small manageable pieces of work and assess how they perform.
>
> *(nurse facilitator)*

Lesson 2: Get to know the people you are working with and their local context

The second lesson relates to developing a sound understanding of the people and the place where you are working to try and facilitate change. This helps to build relationships with the intended recipients of the change process and to get a better sense of the local contextual factors that might influence implementation. Both formal and informal assessments of the context are useful to undertake.

> It is important to conduct site visits and immerse yourself within your implementation context. This provides you with a vital understanding of the people and environments that you are working with, and helps you diagnose their barriers to change. I found it surprising how different general practices are one to the next. Likewise, when I began facilitating I didn't have any experience of the subject area, but I never pretended to practices that I knew something when I didn't. Instead, I made sure I was honest and said I would go and find out something about the evidence if I didn't know, and then made sure I was responsive about returning the evidence to them and where it had come from.
>
> *(KTA 1)*

> When starting work as a facilitator on a brand new project it can often feel like a lot of time with participants can often be spent talking about topics which bear little direct relation to the project. This can often feel frustrating and a bit of a 'waste of time'. However, this is often time well-invested as it functions to help facilitators to build valuable and trusting relationships with participants and enable an informal assessment of the practice context, allowing future facilitation strategies to be tailored accordingly.
>
> *(KTA 2)*

Alongside this informal assessment of the context, it is also helpful to undertake a more formal assessment of the local context, using one of the existing tools and frameworks that are available. In the CKD project, we used two frameworks to assess the local context: the PARIHS sub-elements of context (culture, leadership and orientation towards learning and evaluation) and Bate and colleagues' six core challenges in organising for improvement (Bate et al., 2008). These helped to build up a more detailed picture of the likely barriers during implementation and informed where and how facilitation strategies needed to be tailored.

> Analyse [the] context before you go in and as you progress – you definitely need to understand politics, staffing capabilities around IT, leadership and team culture and you need to have a clear framework for diagnosing blocks and problems and then designing and testing solutions.
>
> *(clinical lead)*

Lesson 3: Find ways to get the work done and keep the project 'on the radar'

Healthcare teams are busy and frequently managing competing priorities. The implementation project may be just one of these many priorities; therefore, the facilitator needs to find ways to keep the staff interested and committed over the long term.

A key role of a facilitator is to keep an improvement project 'on the radar'. In a busy and demanding healthcare environment, even for people with the best intentions, it can be easy for a quality improvement project to become 'just another thing' they haven't got around to doing. Frequently, there is a flurry of activity following a facilitation meeting, but this can quickly tail off as other work takes over and the project works reaches the bottom of their growing 'to-do' list. As a facilitator, it is important to keep in routine contact with staff to monitor and assess progress and, at its most simple, to remind them about the project and to prompt them to complete the tasks they indicated they would do. In this sense, following a facilitation meeting, it's always useful to share (perhaps via email) an agreed list of actions to be completed before you next meet, as this can serve as an aide memoire and enable you to refer to them in future.

(KTA 2)

However, this does not mean actually completing the agreed project actions on behalf of the practice-based improvement team in an attempt to keep things moving:

> BUT . . . as tempting as it can be, it is important not to do any of the project work for participants, but support them in doing it themselves. While this may mean that it takes longer to achieve your project aims, it is fundamental to ensuring the long-term sustainability of any changes made.
>
> *(KTA 2)*

Or becoming too despondent as a facilitator that things are not happening as agreed:

> Often people promise to do things with the best will in the world but don't get them done as quickly as planned . . . or at all. Sometimes it felt a little disappointing when facilitating because you would leave a meeting feeling that everyone was engaged and keen to get on with all of the work that you agreed between then and your return, and everyone was confident that it could be achieved. However, frequently you would go back to a practice and find that little, or nothing, had been done in that time, and that people had sometimes forgotten what it was they were meant to have done, so you ended up feeling that the previous meeting had been a waste and you were going to have to repeat it all again.
>
> *(KTA 1)*

In these situations, the facilitator's job is to try and understand what is going on, pinpoint the underlying causes and help to find practical solutions:

> In most cases people's reasons for not completing things are genuine enough, and facilitation then became about diagnosing any underlying factors that might have led to the failure to complete actions (in addition to reasons that they may have provided) and thinking about how to help them navigate around these problems to avoid a repeat (be that there is a resource/staff imbalance at the practice, not understanding the evidence, differing professional opinions, allocated time or time management).
>
> *(KTA 1)*

It's about identifying a nurse who is struggling as she has no time available and perhaps as the facilitator speaking to the practice manager about some protected time or identifying any other staff members that can be involved.

(nurse facilitator)

Lesson 4: Being organised and planning ahead

Part of keeping the project on the radar involves the facilitator thinking ahead and using project management skills to structure and organise implementation meetings and activities.

> The environment that we operate in for this project can be quite chaotic, dynamic and disorganised. Because time is quite precious in primary care, you can expect that meetings will be moved at short notice quite frequently; people will forget that you are coming, and it can take a long time to get responses from people once you are outside the practice walls. Therefore, I started to prepare for meetings as best as possible to mitigate the risk of these problems. For instance, I began preparing meeting notes prior to a meeting to outline all of the things I needed to cover in that meeting, researched and noted any key bits from previous meetings that needed to be followed up, and most importantly, I always made sure I had my next meeting booked in before I left the practice. Otherwise you would walk out and the date you had in mind would slip by at least a week or two. Then, I wrote up my meeting notes as soon as was practicable so that I didn't forget anything. Another anecdotal comment I received frequently was that 'we got this done because we knew you were coming back in two weeks' so clearly communicating the next meeting date to the whole practice team before leaving avoided any doubt and helped them coordinate their work immediately.
>
> *(KTA 1)*

> Make [the meetings] at the most convenient time to the practice . . . [Think about issues such as] . . . do the staff have allocated admin time? Are they able to block time out to meet with us? Always get a next meeting booked before leaving the practice this is vital otherwise we have found that you can struggle to get back in.
>
> *(nurse facilitator)*

Lesson 5: Be flexible; do not rigidly stick to the initial project plan

Another lesson relates to the need for facilitators to be responsive and adaptable. Even though there is a clear project plan and the facilitator is using project management skills to keep things moving forwards, they need to be flexible and adjust their approach if the situation calls for it. For example, some teams did not find the PDSA approach particularly helpful for all of the issues they were trying to address. In these cases, it was important to work with their concerns and find alternative ways to help them address the collaborative aims, rather than rigidly sticking with the PDSA method.

> PDSAs aren't the answer to everything; don't be afraid of going 'off piste' and design tailor-made approaches so long as they are aligned to aim.
>
> *(clinical lead)*

Lesson 6: Cross-pollinate ideas

When a facilitator is working in several sites at the same time, they can usefully function as a 'knowledge broker' and 'boundary spanner', sharing ideas about things that work well and enabling the spread of best practice.

> We found that practices quite often operate not necessarily in isolation, but frequently not sharing ideas of good practice. We could bridge some of those gaps by bringing suggestions into meetings that we had learnt from facilitating at other practices. This was especially useful in phase 1 as the disparate spacing of the of the practices geographically meant that there wasn't the pre-existing 'communities of practice'.
>
> *(KTA 1)*

Lesson 7: Reinforce the benefits and achievements

To invest time and energy into an improvement project, busy staff need to see 'what's in it for us'; in other words, what benefits will the project bring for them personally, for their practice and for their patients. The facilitator has a role to play in highlighting the potential benefits and demonstrating the achievements made as the project progresses. This helps to keep staff motivated and engaged.

> Reinforce the benefits to the practice [for example]: improved patient care and better health outcomes; staff will have increased knowledge, understanding and better management of their CKD patients; improved patient compliance with better understanding of their condition; appropriate and early referrals to secondary care; less referrals to secondary care; being involved can be used for appraisal/PDP . . . [also what the practice is getting for free, such as] . . . CKD/IMPAKT Improvement Guide; educational events; facilitation at practice visits and 1:1 education/facilitation if requested.
>
> *(nurse facilitator)*

Lesson 8: Try to embed regular project team meetings

For the team involved in facilitating the project, regular communication is essential. This is particularly important in a large project, such as the one we are describing, where several people are members of the project team, with different roles and contributions to make to the overall project aim. Alongside the monthly scheduled project team meetings, we also found it helpful to have short weekly catch-ups where possible to update on progress, identify when problems were occurring and develop real-time solutions for the facilitators. This is likely to be different for individual projects; the main point to make is the need for some form of regular communication and contact.

> Try and embed a weekly meet no matter how brief – healthcare professionals are rubbish at this without a strong guiding hand and some habit formation as the clinical pressures get responded to automatically. Equally you should meet as a facilitator/project team weekly.
>
> *(clinical lead)*

Lesson 9: Communicate, communicate, communicate

From the outset of the project, a clear and comprehensive communication plan is vital to keep the various stakeholders informed and on board with the project. This involves thinking about the types of information different stakeholder groups will find most useful and how best to get the information to them. In our project, this involved strategies for communicating with the senior sponsors, the expert stakeholder group, participating practices and the improvement teams.

> This requires a strategy, a stakeholder map and awareness of preferred communication formats and then multiple delivery methods. Beware this all takes time and energy.
>
> *(clinical lead)*

Lesson 10: Work with a team not an individual

The final lesson relates to who the facilitator works with in the immediate local setting. Although there may be individual champions who are enthusiastic about the project, it is important not to forget about the wider team that need to embrace the proposed changes. This is key to embedding the changes in practice and ensuring sustainability over the longer term.

> Within a clinical environment there can often be one particularly enthusiastic person who is happy and willing to take on all tasks within a project. This can be a great asset, but it's important to ensure that you work with a team of people, not just this one person. This is to ensure that changes are embedded across the team and that any changes made aren't just temporary improvements that disappear if this sole person changes job or department. If this is the case, clinical practice can often end up in a worse place than it began.
>
> *(KTA 2)*

What this case study adds to our overall understanding of facilitation

Dogherty and colleagues make a distinction between the facilitator role and the facilitation process (Dogherty et al., 2010) and we believe that our case study contributes insights to both of these elements. In relation to the facilitator role, we set out working with novice facilitators who were newly appointed to the role, did not have prior experience of healthcare (in the first collaborative) and were required to work with a diverse range of organisations within different local environments. This placed a considerable weight of expectation on the facilitators in terms of developing knowledge and skills in evidence translation, quality improvement, facilitating implementation, change management and working within a primary care environment – all within a relatively short period of time. Whether we would adopt a similar approach again is an interesting point for reflection; however, our experience suggests that if the right people are recruited to the role, it is possible to work with novice facilitators, providing they are placed within a supportive facilitation team structure, where they can acquire learning about the role and access advice and guidance. One advantage that the KTAs brought as external facilitators was that they came from outside the NHS with its institutionalised ways of working and introducing change.

Through a combination of formal and informal mechanisms the experiential learning of facilitators can itself be facilitated, rather than occurring as a process of trial and error, which is what tends to happen when structures are not in place to support the learning process (Harvey et al., 2002). The introduction of a novice clinical facilitator in the second collaborative allowed us to begin exploring the different combinations of facilitator roles and skills. The seconded nurse facilitator clearly brought local knowledge and credibility to the facilitation team. Interestingly, as this facilitator began to develop her knowledge, skills and confidence in the role, the original (novice) facilitators gradually began to move to a more 'hands-off' role – supporting the new facilitator, but working at a more strategic/external role across a number of different projects. This demonstrates the potential for building the type of cascade model of facilitation that was described earlier in the book, which clearly has benefits in relation to the sustainability and spread of evidence-based practice within a local healthcare setting. However, as with the KTAs, it is important to identify internal facilitators with the right attributes, attitudes and skill-set.

In terms of the facilitation process, the improvement collaborative methodology that we adopted helped to address key aspects of the implementation process, such as synthesising the relevant evidence and checking it out with key stakeholders (via an expert faculty), establishing goals, identifying metrics to track progress, guiding action at a local level (through PDSA cycles) and sharing learning and experiences (at the collaborative learning events). In practice, these component elements of the improvement collaborative were seen to act as enablers of implementation, reinforced by the additional element of a practice facilitator. Adding this more active facilitation element allowed us to tailor our approach – particularly in response to specific issues at a local level – rather than sticking rigidly to what is often a 'blueprint' model for improvement collaboratives. We would suggest that having designated facilitators in the collaborative model could help to make the approach more context-sensitive and reduce the inherent variation reported within improvement collaborative projects (Schouten et al., 2008; de Silva, 2014). Within this broad collaborative approach, we also learnt a lot about the practicalities of facilitation, for example, balancing project management skills with flexibility and responsiveness. In turn, this depends upon a sound understanding of the local practice context and good relationships with the staff involved.

On a final note, we recognise that there is still more to discover about facilitation and facilitators in order to reduce the variations in processes and outcomes. Some questions that we would suggest need further exploration include the following: Do all teams require the same level of facilitation input? How can the dose and frequency of facilitation be adjusted according to local needs and circumstances? What is the ideal combination of facilitator characteristics and skills (clinical versus non-clinical; seniority versus experience; internal versus external)? Is it better to pre-define objectives and measures for improvement (as in the collaborative model) or to allow local teams to define their aims and related metrics? These are some of the questions that we are continuing to explore in our ongoing programmes of work.

References

Bate, P., Mendel, P. & Robert, G. 2008. *Organising for Quality: The Improvement Journeys of Leading Hospitals in Europe and the United States*. Abingdon: Radcliffe.

De Silva, D. 2014. *Improvement Collaboratives in Health Care: Evidence Scan*. London: The Health Foundation.

Dogherty, E.J., Harrison, M.B. & Graham, I.D. 2010. Facilitation as a role and process in achieving evidence-based practice in nursing: a focused review of concept and meaning. *Worldviews on Evidence Based Nursing*, 7, 76–89.

Go, A.S., Chertow, G.M., Fan, D., McCulloch, C.E. & Hsu, C.Y. 2004. Chronic kidney disease and the risks of death, cardiovascular events, and hospitalization. *New England Journal of Medicine*, 351, 1296–305.

Grimshaw, J.M., Thomas, R.E., Maclennan, G., Fraser, C., Ramsay, C.R., Vale, L., et al. 2004. Effectiveness and efficiency of guideline dissemination and implementation strategies. *Health Technology Assessment*, 8, iii–iv, 1–72.

Harvey, G., Loftus-Hills, A., Rycroft-Malone, J., Titchen, A., Kitson, A., McCormack, B. & Seers, K. 2002. Getting evidence into practice: the role and function of facilitation. *Journal of Advanced Nursing*, 37, 577–88.

Harvey, G., Fitzgerald, L., Fielden, S., McBride, A., Waterman, H., Bamford, D., Kislov, R. & Boaden, R. 2011. The NIHR collaboration for leadership in applied health research and care (CLAHRC) for Greater Manchester: combining empirical, theoretical and experiential evidence to design and evaluate a large-scale implementation strategy. *Implementation Science*, 6, 96.

Humphreys, J., Harvey, G., Coleiro, M., Butler, B., Barclay, A., Gwozdziewicz, M., O'Donoghue, D. & Hegarty, J. 2012. A collaborative project to improve identification and management of patients with chronic kidney disease in a primary care setting in Greater Manchester. *BMJ Quality & Safety*, 21, 700–708.

IHI (Institute for Healthcare Improvement) 2003. *The Breakthrough Series: IHI's Collaborative Model for Achieving Breakthrough Improvement*. IHI Innovation Series white paper. Boston, MA: Institute for Healthcare Improvement.

IMPAKT™ 2013. *A Guide to Using IMPAKT™ to Improve Diagnosis and Care for People with Chronic Kidney Disease* [Online]. http://clahrc-gm.nihr.ac.uk/cms/wp-content/uploads/IMPAKT-CKD-Improvement-Guide.pdf. University Hospitals of Leicester NHS Trust [accessed 16 June 2014].

K/DOQI 2002. Clinical practice guidelines for chronic kidney disease. Evaluation, classification and stratification. *American Journal of Kidney Diseases*, 39, S17–S31.

Kitson, A., Harvey, G. & McCormack, B. 1998. Enabling the implementation of evidence based practice: a conceptual framework. *Quality in Health Care*, 7, 149–58.

Langley, G.J., Nolan, K.M., Norman, C.L., Provost, L.P. & Nolan, T.W. 1996. *The Improvement Guide. A Practical Guide to Enhancing Organisational Performance*. San Francisco, CA: Jossey-Bass.

McCormack, B., Kitson, A., Harvey, G., Rycroft-Malone, J., Titchen, A. & Seers, K. 2002. Getting evidence into practice: the meaning of 'context'. *Journal of Advanced Nursing*, 38, 94–104.

NICE (National Institute for Health and Clinical Excellence) 2008. *Chronic Kidney Disease: National Clinical Guideline for Early Identification and Management in Adults in Primary and Secondary Care*. London: National Institute for Health and Clinical Excellence.

Øvretveit, J., Bate, P., Cleary, P., Cretin, S., Gustafson, D., McInnes, K., et al. 2002. Quality collaboratives: lessons from research. *Quality and Safety in Health Care*, 11, 345–51.

Rothwell, K., Harvey, G. & Humphreys, J. 2012. *Qualitative Evaluation of the Chronic Kidney Disease (CKD) Improvement Project*. Manchester: NIHR CLAHRC for Greater Manchester.

Rycroft-Malone, J., Kitson, A., Harvey, G., McCormack, B., Seers, K., Titchen, A. & Estabrooks, C. 2002. Ingredients for change: revisiting a conceptual framework. *Quality and Safety in Health Care*, 11, 174–80.

Schouten, L.M.T., Hulscher, M.E.J.L., Everdingen, J.J.E.V., Huijsman, R. & Grol, R.P.T.M. 2008. Evidence for the impact of quality improvement collaboratives: systematic review. *British Medical Journal*, 336, 1491–4.

Stevens, P.E., O'Donoghue, D.J., De Lusignan, S., Van Vlymen, J., Klebe, B., Middleton, R., et al. 2007. Chronic kidney disease management in the United Kingdom: NEOERICA project results. *Kidney International*, 72, 92–9.

9

A FACILITATION PROJECT TO IMPROVE THE MANAGEMENT OF CONTINENCE IN EUROPEAN NURSING HOMES

Gill Harvey and Alison Kitson

Introduction and background to the facilitation project

This case study presents a project undertaken as part of a European research study to compare two different approaches to facilitating the implementation of evidence-based recommendations for managing continence in a long-term nursing care setting. The research study – titled 'Facilitating Implementation of Research Evidence' (FIRE) – was undertaken as a pragmatic randomised controlled trial with funding from the European Union and took place between 2008 and 2013 (Seers et al., 2012). The trial had three arms: arm 1 received standard dissemination of evidence-based recommendations for continence care along with a PowerPoint presentation on implementation; arm 2 received the standard dissemination plus a goal-centred approach to facilitation; in arm 3, the same standard dissemination was accompanied by an emancipatory model of facilitation.

In this chapter, we will describe the experience of designing and facilitating the strategy that was applied in arm 2 of the trial. This approach to facilitation was based upon similar ideas and principles of facilitation that we have outlined in earlier chapters of the book. It started with the evidence to be implemented (in this case, a series of recommendations for managing continence) and applied improvement methods and thinking alongside organisational theories of change to identify goals for implementation, agree ways of monitoring progress against the goals and undertake cycles of action and evaluation to implement the agreed changes. By contrast, the facilitation approach in arm 3 of the study adopted an approach to facilitation based upon theories of critical social science. The emphasis here was on inquiry and development at the level of individuals and the culture and context in which they were working, with the aim of enabling emancipatory action to overcome barriers to implementation (Manley and McCormack, 2003; McCormack et al., 2013).

We begin the chapter by outlining the background to the study, including how the focus of specific implementation and facilitation activities was identified. We then describe how we applied our approach to facilitating implementation, including both the facilitator roles and the facilitation strategies that were employed to identify and work towards agreed goals, engage key stakeholders and address the contextual issues. Key areas to be highlighted include the experience of working with an external–internal model of facilitation and using virtual methods to facilitate local projects and support internal facilitators who were based in different countries throughout Europe. Formative evaluation data relating to the processes and outcomes of implementation will be presented before we conclude the chapter by reflecting on the lessons we learnt about facilitation during the study, including what we think this adds to the knowledge base about facilitation in relation to evidence-based healthcare.

The FIRE study

The initial idea for the FIRE study arose from the experience of developing, applying and refining the PARIHS (Promoting Action on Research Implementation in Health Services) framework. Although our own and others' experiences suggested a level of face and content validity for PARIHS, questions remained about the relationships between different elements and sub-elements of the model and about how to apply facilitation to operationalise PARIHS within an implementation project (Kitson et al., 2008; Helfrich et al., 2010). Of particular interest was the question of whether a 'good enough' model of facilitation existed? Given the continuum of facilitation presented in the PARIHS concept analysis (Harvey et al., 2002), was it possible to determine a point on the continuum that provided a sufficient 'dose' of facilitation to support the implementation of research evidence into practice? These questions subsequently informed the design of the FIRE study and the specific aim it set out to address, namely to evaluate the feasibility, effectiveness and cost-effectiveness of two different models of facilitation in promoting the uptake of research evidence on continence management. As outlined in the introduction to the chapter, two different models of facilitation were developed and tested within the study, each

> requiring different levels of facilitator skills and knowledge and the application of different methods of implementation, with corresponding different levels of resource requirements in terms of preparation and support of facilitators and the ways in which they work with individuals and teams who are attempting to implement research into practice.
>
> *(Seers et al., 2012, p.3)*

Of specific interest in this chapter are the methods and processes used to develop and implement the goal-focused model of facilitation (arm 2) and how this approach to facilitation worked in practice.

The study was conducted in long-term nursing care settings in four countries: Sweden, Ireland, England and the Netherlands. In some countries, these were residential nursing homes, in others they were hospitals with beds for long-term care of older people (aged over 60). In each country, two sites were allocated to each of the three study arms, resulting in a total of 24 long-term nursing care facilities participating in the study. In arm 2 of the study there were eight sites: two from each of the four countries involved in the FIRE study.

The evidence base

The evidence to be implemented was derived from guidelines that were developed by the Fourth International Consultation on Incontinence (DuBeau et al., 2009) and specifically the algorithm produced by a working committee that examined the research evidence relating to incontinence in frail older people. This evidence was reviewed by continence experts on the

FIRE project advisory board and by experts in each of the four countries participating in the study to ensure its relevance at a national level. Following this process, it was agreed that the focus of implementation in the FIRE study would be on four evidence-based recommendations relating to active screening for urinary incontinence, detailed assessment, individualised treatment plans and specialist referral as needed. These recommendations, along with the more detailed criteria relating to each recommendation, formed the starting point for implementation in all of the study sites.

Overview of the facilitation approach

The project explicitly adopted an external–internal model of facilitation. Two members of the FIRE project team (GH and AK) were designated the role of external facilitators, with the remit of designing a facilitation intervention to be applied in arm 2 of the trial and then preparing and supporting internal facilitators to work with this facilitation intervention. Before describing the design and application of the facilitation strategy, we will outline how the internal facilitators were selected from the sites engaged in the FIRE study.

Recruitment of internal facilitators

Recruitment of internal facilitators commenced once sites that had agreed to participate in the FIRE study had been allocated to one of the three study arms. However, prior to signing up to participate in the research, all prospective sites were provided with a summary of the type of people that would be required to take on an internal facilitator role if their organisation was allocated to arms 2 or 3 of the study. The summary listed the essential criteria that the study team felt were essential to take on a facilitator role, based on previous research and experiences of working with the role in practice (Box 9.1).

BOX 9.1 CRITERIA FOR SELECTING INTERNAL FACILITATORS

When selecting an internal facilitator, we are looking for someone who:

- Has some knowledge of good practice in continence care and has an interest in the topic (has a positive attitude towards evidence and how evidence can help develop this aspect of patient/resident care and can demonstrate some essential knowledge of continence promotion and key aspects of best practice in continence management, e.g. assessment, use of continence aids)
- Knows co-workers (has been in the organisation long enough to know the staff and how they work)
- Knows the environment (has some insight into the culture of the setting)
- Knows the organisation (knows their way around the organisation, e.g. who's who, policies in place, decision-making structures)
- Occupies a clinical leadership position (one where they have authority or are able to negotiate authority to make decisions about practice; how practice is organised; resources impacting on practice)

- Possesses effective communication skills (could include attributes of being open minded, being creative, has experience of managing meetings/groups, able to talk in front of groups)
- Is self-aware and resilient (has insight into their support needs, but is also not afraid of challenge/conflict; willing to engage in own professional development)
- Is reliable and dependable (has time they can dedicate to this work [in writing from their manager]; carries through with responsibilities, meets deadlines or negotiates otherwise; is not intending to be on extended leave during intervention period)

Members of the FIRE project research team discussed the criteria with senior managers in the sites, for example, nursing home managers, who were then asked to nominate the individual they would like to take on the internal facilitator role. It was also suggested that a 'buddy' role be identified to provide additional support and cover for the internal facilitator as needed (Box 9.2).

BOX 9.2 CRITERIA FOR FACILITATOR BUDDIES

- Prepared to work with and help the local facilitator for the duration of the project
- Willing to step in to attend the training programme in the event that the nominated facilitator is unable to attend
- Prepared to read the material and help interpret the contents, working closely with the facilitator
- Willing to act as a support to the facilitator
- Able to provide feedback to the facilitator about the process
- Willing to help the facilitator get the project up and running
- Prepared to help with dissemination

At the end of this process – and following the allocation of two nursing home facilities in each country to arm 2 of the study – eight internal facilitators were identified and some sites also had agreed facilitator buddies. All eight internal facilitators were invited to a three-day residential programme, which formed the starting point of the facilitation intervention.

Elements of the facilitation strategy

The design of the research study meant that the two external facilitators had to prepare and support eight internal facilitators all working in different organisations across four European countries. To manage this complexity, the facilitation strategy involved a combination of face-to-face and virtual working. The external facilitators began by designing the facilitation approach to be adopted in the study (the details of which are outlined in the following section) and used this to plan an initial three-day development programme for internal facilitators.

The FIRE research protocol effectively specified the 'dose' of facilitation that would be provided in arms 2 and 3 of the study, including the overall timeframe for the intervention, the length of the initial development programme and the subsequent frequency and amount of support to be provided to the internal facilitators. In arm 2, the overall length of the intervention was 12 months, with the initial three-day training and development programme, followed by monthly 90-minute teleconferences between the external and internal facilitators. (The more intensive nature of the arm 3 intervention was reflected in a longer total intervention period and a five-day development programme for internal facilitators.)

The development programme for internal facilitators took place in May 2010. This was a residential programme, which was held in one of the participating countries, the Netherlands. In line with the PARIHS framework and the goal-focused model of facilitation, the programme addressed key areas such as understanding and interpreting evidence within a local context, planning and structuring the implementation process (establishing goals and measures, monitoring progress and taking action to improve) and the facilitator role and methods. A mixture of large group presentation and small group interactive learning approaches were used, taking particular account of the language issues for internal facilitators who did not have English as their first language. Translators from Sweden and Netherlands were present throughout the residential programme to provide assistance to the internal facilitators where required and key documentation to be used in the study was also translated into the relevant language. All the internal facilitators were provided with a facilitation learning resource, which contained the materials used during the learning programme, along with other useful information and contact details.

At the end of the residential programme, a timetable for the monthly teleconference meetings for the following year was agreed. These took place at the same time on the same day of the month, allowing the internal facilitators to plan them into their diaries. Internal facilitators were encouraged to involve their buddies in the teleconference. Each call was scheduled for 90 minutes and followed a similar agenda, commencing with a review of the notes from the previous meeting and any matters arising. This was followed by an update from individual sites, including a review of progress against the agreed goals, feedback on internal audit data and a discussion of any particular problems or challenges the internal facilitator was facing. Although the meeting was chaired by one of the external facilitators, internal facilitators were encouraged to share experiences and offer solutions relating to their fellow internal facilitators' experiences and perceived barriers to implementation. On different occasions, there was also specialist input into the meetings, for example, from continence experts or in relation to the audit programme that was being used. The meeting concluded with an evaluation process, where all participants were asked to reflect on how they felt the meeting had gone and suggestions for how it could be improved next time around. Following the meeting, action notes were circulated along with reflections from the external facilitators regarding key learning points and issues for consideration to be discussed at the subsequent teleconference.

In order to support the time needed to carry out the internal facilitator role, there was provision in the FIRE budget to fund the equivalent of 19 days of protected time for each of the internal facilitators (10 days to work on the implementation and evaluation of the evidence-based recommendations; 3 days for the residential training; 12 half days for monthly teleconferences). The external facilitators were each funded for 16 days over the year to fulfil their role.

At the end of the 12 months, a closing meeting was held in Sweden. The internal facilitators and their buddies were invited to attend this meeting which took place over a 24-hour period. Each facilitator/buddy was asked to prepare a short presentation on the achievements from the project within their own organisation. This was followed by a session in which the internal facilitators, the buddies and the external facilitators all reflected on the experience of the project, the facilitation role and process and the lessons learnt. Subsequent sessions addressed ideas and plans for maintaining and spreading improvement and disseminating the learning from the project.

Implementing the evidence: project design

The methods used to address the challenge of translating the evidence-based recommendations for continence care closely reflect the model of facilitation we have outlined so far in the book – not surprising as we had the role of external facilitators for the intervention! Within the three-day residential programme, we worked with the internal facilitators to review the recommendations and criteria relating to screening, assessment, individualised care and referral and think about how these aligned in terms of current policy and practice in their own organisations. Although some were already practising in ways that were consistent with some or all of the recommendations, others were not; however, there was consensus amongst the internal facilitators that they wanted to aim for 100% compliance to all of the recommendations within the 12-month timeframe of the intervention. Measures to monitor progress towards the aims were also specified in the form of audit criteria; 16 in total (Box 9.3). (Note: These criteria were identified for the purpose of internal audit. Process and outcome data were collected independently within the care setting as part of the trial.)

BOX 9.3   AGREED AIMS AND AUDIT CRITERIA FOR IMPLEMENTING THE EVIDENCE-BASED RECOMMENDATIONS

Recommendation 1: Each patient/resident has been actively screened for symptoms of urinary incontinence (UI)

Agreed compliance: 100%
Audit criteria:

1.1 Each resident has a documented record of their continence history
1.2 The continence history includes detailed information about the bladder habits of the resident
1.3 The continence history includes information about the resident's medical condition that may affect their ability to be continent

Recommendation 2: A detailed assessment is carried out which includes an assessment of co-morbid conditions, full urinalysis, wet checks to assess frequency and type of UI specified

Agreed compliance: 100%

(continued)

(continued)

Audit criteria:

2.1 Each resident who has been identified as having UI has a documented record of their continence assessment
2.2 The continence assessment includes a detailed consideration of relevant factors that might influence the resident's ability to be continent, both during the day and at night
2.3 The assessment includes a frequency volume chart
2.4 The assessment includes an indication of the type of UI

Recommendation 3: An individual treatment plan should be in place for setting individual goals for each resident with UI, working with residents' treatment preferences, explicit bladder retraining programmes and linking the treatment plan to the resident's overall quality of life

Agreed compliance: 100%
Audit criteria:

3.1 There is an individualised treatment plan for every resident with UI
3.2 The plan includes review dates
3.3 The plan is up to date at the time of audit
3.4 Relevant methods of management are documented as being used
3.5 There is documented evidence that the resident/representative has been involved in developing the plan of care for managing their UI
3.6 There is documented evidence of active intervention for those residents where indicated in the assessment

Recommendation 4: Specialist referral should be made where required

Agreed compliance: 100%
Audit criteria:

4.1 Residents who require specialist referral get referred to the appropriate specialist
4.2 Residents' care plans document the reasons for the referral
4.3 Residents' care plans document the outcome of the referral

In order to help manage the audit process and because the facilitators were geographically spread, we opted to use an electronic audit system developed by the Joanna Briggs Institute (JBI). This system – the Practical Application of Evidence System (PACES) – would allow internal facilitators to enter audit data online and the results could then be analysed, compared and fed back electronically. An initial introduction to the PACES system was provided at the residential programme. The agreed audit criteria were then loaded into PACES and all the internal facilitators were given access to the system, with guidance on how to use it. Further technical support was provided on the use of PACES at the monthly teleconferences via a member of staff at JBI who was involved in developing and running PACES.

Alongside the strategies that were used to interpret the evidence and translate it into measurable goals and criteria, other activities that formed part of the facilitation approach included various assessments of the local context and perceived barriers to implementation. This involved identifying key stakeholders and how they might support or hinder the implementation process. At a personal level, internal facilitators reflected on their own experiences of facilitation and of being facilitated to identify essential characteristics of effective facilitation and explore the relationships between facilitation and leadership (in a similar process to that described in Chapter 5). In preparing to start the implementation project within their own organisation, the internal facilitators were encouraged to establish a small implementation team that would meet regularly to plan, action and evaluate agreed changes using approaches such as Plan–Do–Study–Act cycles. A template for an implementation plan was provided by the external facilitators, highlighting the key areas that needed to be taken into consideration at a local level, both in relation to specific implementation activities such as audit and action cycles and broader issues of stakeholder engagement and communication (Figure 9.1).

Methods used to identify and work with stakeholders

A discussion around stakeholder engagement and communication took place during the internal facilitator development programme and ideas were exchanged about ways to do this.

FiRE

Facilitating Implementation
of Research Evidence

PROJECT PLAN FOR ....

The Overall Project Aims:	

Situational Analysis:
  – Contextual Factors
  – Scope of Project
  – Relevance of topic	

Key Stakeholders:
  – Who?
  – Why?	

Improvement Team:
  – Members
  – Meetings (when, where, how often)	

Baseline Audit Data Collection: – Who, when and where?	

Action Plan:
  – Tests of change: 1st
                       2nd
                       3rd	

Communication Plan: – Who, what, how often?	

FIGURE 9.1 Template for local implementation plan

One activity undertaken by the internal facilitators during the residential programme was to design a poster that they could customise and then display within their local care setting to inform colleagues and residents about the project. Once they returned back to their own organisations it was very much up to the internal facilitators to follow through their plans for engaging with the key stakeholders they had identified, often working alongside their buddy. Different facilitators approached this in different ways. Many of them made presentations to their colleagues following the residential course to explain the project and what they were try-ing to achieve. Some stakeholders were particularly influential in different countries. For exam-ple, in Sweden the specialist nurses working for incontinence product companies traditionally played an important educational role for staff within nursing home facilities. This posed some challenges for the internal facilitators, for example, in terms of persuading their colleagues to think in terms of 'continence', rather than selecting the best products to manage incontinence.

Methods used to assess and respond to contextual issues

Assessment of the local context for implementation began at the residential programme and continued as a regular discussion item at the monthly teleconference meetings. The facilita-tors did not use a formal context assessment instrument, but were encouraged to reflect on the PARIHS dimensions of culture, leadership and organisational learning/evaluation when planning and reviewing their implementation plans. For many of the internal facilitators, there was a need to change the mindset within the organisation about the potential to achieve con-tinence with some of their long-term residents and clients. This presented a significant barrier to implementation. When this became apparent during the monthly teleconference meetings, the external facilitators arranged for a continence nurse specialist who was a member of the project advisory group to attend the next teleconference meeting. This proved very successful and provided the internal facilitators with a range of practical advice, ideas and resources that they could use within the local setting. In one organisation, the internal facilitator and buddy undertook a series of interviews with residents to explore their experiences of incontinence; these resident stories proved to be very powerful in getting the message across about what it was like to live with incontinence and helped to engage their colleagues with the project.

The support from local leaders and managers proved to be an important factor in terms of the facilitators' ability to address contextual barriers, particularly as a number of the organisa-tions were experiencing major re-organisation, including new ownership arrangements and management restructuring. This, in turn, related to the facilitator's position in the organisation and their level of authority and confidence to fulfil the role. In some sites, the facilitator was also the unit manager; in this situation, the facilitator could use their designated authority to develop and introduce new documentation, such as continence screening and assessment tools. However, in another setting, the internal facilitator was less qualified than the registered nurses who held the overall responsibility for resident care. Despite the fact that this facilitator had the senior manager as her buddy, she found it very difficult to gain commitment to the project within the nursing home and did not feel that she had the authority to suggest or introduce some of the changes that were required.

In some countries, things happening at the wider contextual level also had a bearing on implementation, particularly the role of external inspection and regulatory bodies. Where inspections of long-term care facilities were taking place and included a focus on continence care, this provided an opportunity for the facilitators to align what they were doing as part of the FIRE project to the regulatory standards the organisation was required to meet. This was a particularly useful way to raise the profile of the project with more senior managers and to gain their attention and support.

Evaluating the impact of facilitation

Throughout (and before and beyond) the intervention period, data collection was ongoing in each of the eight organisations where the internal facilitators worked. Data relating to the processes and outcomes of continence care, the organisational context and the facilitation process were gathered by researchers who were independent of the external facilitators and the facilitation intervention. These data informed the overall evaluation strategy of the FIRE project and were collected at baseline and then over a period of 24 months; however, these data were not available to either the external or internal facilitators during the course of the intervention. In terms of assessing the impact of the intervention in real time, the main data sources were the internal audit conducted by the facilitators as part of the facilitation intervention, the feedback gained during the monthly teleconferences and the external facilitators' ongoing reflections on the process. Further feedback was also collated at the final project meeting at the end of the intervention period. We will summarise these data to report the processes and outcomes of the facilitation intervention. Detailed analysis and reporting of the main trial findings is in progress at the time of writing; therefore, we will not be passing any judgement on the relative effectiveness of type A or type B facilitation. Rather, our intention here is to describe what we learnt from our own formative evaluation of type A facilitation.

Internal evaluation of impact

As described, agreement on the criteria to be measured and the aims in terms of compliance was reached at the facilitator development programme (see Box 9.3). The original plan was to undertake a full baseline audit against all 16 criteria and then commence action cycles for one recommendation at a time, followed by a repeat audit. The purpose of the staged approach to acting on the baseline audit data was to make the process more manageable as most of the internal facilitators had very little experience of audit and none had used an electronic system such as PACES. Furthermore, a number of the facilitators lacked confidence and experience of using information technology (IT), while others had the challenge of working in a second language. Although PACES was selected to try and make the audit process easier, the facilitators' starting position (in terms of little prior experience of audit and/or limited IT skills) effectively meant that for some PACES created an additional complicated step in the implementation process, particularly in terms of some of the specifications required to use PACES (Harvey et al., 2012). Collectively, these issues presented a significant barrier to progress in terms of the baseline audit. In order to deal with the problems the facilitators were facing, a number of solutions were introduced: to simplify the baseline audit, the guideline recommendations were taken one at a time, starting with recommendation 1 and working towards recommendation 4 in a sequential process; the facilitators were given the option to undertake a paper-based audit and submit the data to the PACES coordinator for inputting; some of the activities required to use PACES were undertaken by the external facilitators and the PACES coordinator.

These modifications produced both intended and unintended consequences. The internal facilitators felt less daunted by the prospect of undertaking the audit and had mostly commenced the audit process by months 4–5 of the project. By the end of the 12-month intervention period, seven of the eight sites had audited recommendations 1 and 2 and four sites had audited all of the recommendations; however, none of the sites had undertaken a re-audit. (Note: One of the eight sites involved in the intervention participated very little in the project following attendance at the residential programme and did not actively engage with the internal audit process.) Reducing the scale of the task the facilitators had to undertake was important in terms of feasibility and confidence building, although from the perspective of the external facilitators, it meant that it was not possible to get a true baseline measure of practice. Once local teams began to look at the results from the audit of recommendation 1, they started to discuss and introduce changes that also affected the other recommendations relating to assessment and care planning. For example, if the audit of screening (recommendation 1) showed potential for improvement, this invariably led to wider discussions about continence assessment tools and testing these tools out when planning the care of individual patients. Consequently the audit data cannot be interpreted as an accurate measure of baseline performance; rather they served as a useful catalyst to stimulate action at a local level by highlighting the potential for improvement. In this respect, there was considerable variation amongst the different sites (see Table 9.1), so although some sites may have initiated action prior to measuring compliance, they still had significant scope to improve.

Despite the challenges of learning the audit process, it was clear by the half-way point of the intervention that the internal facilitators were beginning to use the data to engage in discussion with colleagues and feedback to their managers. In this way, the audit data played an important role in focusing discussions around the evidence and creating a commitment to introduce changes, such as trialling new assessment documentation.

Feedback from monthly teleconferences (including external facilitators' reflections)

A total of 12 teleconference meetings were held. Attendance at these meetings was variable; some organisations were represented at all the meetings, others at relatively few. Some internal facilitators attended most of the meetings with their buddy; other internal facilitators did not involve the buddy at all. During the course of the intervention, two internal facilitators had to take time off work due to ill-health. In one case, the buddy stepped in to take over the internal facilitator role; in the other case, a new facilitator was identified and one of the external facilitators provided a shorter (two-day) version of the facilitator development programme for the new internal facilitator and her buddy. Table 9.2 summarises the pattern of attendance at teleconference meetings by site. This suggests that within the study, two sites had a high level of engagement with the intervention and two had a low level of engagement. The remaining four sites had a medium to high level of engagement (taking into account that one of these sites started the project five months later than planned).

Analysis of the notes of the teleconference discussions – and the external facilitators' reflections on the meetings – reveals a number of key themes. First, issues within the local context presented obstacles to the internal facilitators that tended to slow down their progress with implementing the project plans they had developed. These obstacles included day-to-day events such as having to work shift systems and the impact of vacation periods, alongside

TABLE 9.1 Self-reported compliance to internal audit criteria by site (%)

Audit criteria	Site 1	Site 2	Site 3	Site 4	Site 5	Site 6	Site 7	Average
Recommendation 1: Screening								
1.1 Documented history	95	100	24	100	100	95	100	89
1.2 Detailed information on bladder habits	5	100	4	100	100	9	60	56
1.3 Relevant information about medical condition	5	100	4	0	100	2	76	58
Recommendation 2: Assessment								
2.1 Documented assessment	91	50	93	100	100	32	100	87
2.2 Detailed consideration of relevant factors	5	0	0	0	67	26	100	36
2.3 Frequency volume chart	30	35	90	0	45	6	82	41
2.4 Indication of type of urinary incontinence	58	80	93	76	67	26	100	70
Recommendation 3: Individualised care plan								
3.1 Individualised treatment plan	60	Not audited	56	Not audited	100	89	Not audited	79
3.2 Includes review dates	100		0		100	64		77
3.3 Plan up to date	75		0		100	75		71
3.4 Relevant management methods	100		14		100	82		82
3.5 Evidence of resident involvement	60		0		100	79		67
3.6 Active intervention	14		0		100	54		50
Recommendation 4: Specialist referral								
4.1 Referral where required	100	Not audited	Not audited	Not audited	100	100	Not audited	100
4.2 Documented reason for referral	100				0	0		33
4.3 Outcome documented	100				0	0		33

organisational level events such as re-organisation and new management, other projects coming on stream and visits from external inspectorates. Second, the difficulty of getting to grips with the audit process and using the PACES system tended to overshadow the discussion in a number of the early meetings. Consequently, some of the facilitators became frustrated, perceiving the audit as something that was potentially getting in the way of them making the changes they wanted to implement. Third, after four or five months – and once the initial problems with the audit were being addressed – the need for technical advice on continence care became apparent. The contribution from a continence nurse specialist at two of the meetings was very beneficial and greatly valued; in the words of one of the internal facilitators, 'it made the guidelines come to life'. Fourth, despite the difficulties and the challenges encountered, the internal facilitators clearly began to develop their own knowledge and understanding of the facilitation process and became increasingly confident in their role. This is particularly reflected in the feedback from the meeting held at the end of the intervention period.

TABLE 9.2 Attendance at teleconference meetings by site

Meeting	Site 1	Site 2	Site 3	Site 4	Site 5	Site 6	Site 7	Site 8
1	IF	IF	IF & B	Late start	IF & B	IF & B	IF	X
2	X	IF & B	IF & B	Late start	IF & B	IF & B	IF	IF & B
3	IF	IF	X	Late start	IF & B	IF & B	X	X
4	IF	IF	IF & B	Late start	IF	IF	X	X
5	IF	X	IF & B	Late start	IF & B	IF & B	IF	IF & B
6	IF	X	IF & B	IF	IF	IF & B	X	X
7	IF	X	IF & B	IF	IF	IF	X	X
8	IF	IF_2	IF_2	X	IF & B	IF & B	X	X
9	IF	IF_2	IF_2	IF & B	IF & B	IF & B	X	X
10	X	IF_2	X	IF	IF	IF & B	X	X
11	X	X	IF_2	IF	IF	IF & B	X	X
12	IF	IF_2	IF_2	X	IF & B	IF	X	B
Total	9	8	10	5	12	12	3	3

Abbreviations: IF, internal facilitator; IF_2, replacement internal facilitator; B, buddy; X, non-attendance.

Source: Late start refers to one organisation that came into the FIRE study later than planned; the intervention continued for a full 12 months with ongoing communication between the external and internal facilitator/buddy

Feedback from the closing meeting

Structured discussion amongst the internal facilitators and buddies at the end of intervention meeting revealed the various challenges they had experienced during the project – some relating to their own perceived level of knowledge and skills, others to issues of language and availability of translation and others to barriers encountered in their own organisations. In terms of learning from the project, key points highlighted in Box 9.4 indicate their increasing awareness of facilitation. As one facilitator commented,

> Being involved in this project has enhanced the continence care of our residents and shown us a new way of learning called facilitation.

BOX 9.4 INTERNAL FACILITATOR (AND BUDDY) REFLECTIONS ON THEIR EXPERIENCE

Key challenges

- Nursing staff resistance to engage
- Team rosters/conflicts
- Multiple projects happening at the same time
- Lack of IT and audit skills

Key learning points

- Benefits of taking things step by step
- Small changes can be effective; usefulness of the Plan–Do–Study–Act model

- Lack of continence expertise
- Needed expert advice earlier in the project
- Novice facilitation skills
- Language difficulties, especially during teleconferences
- All documentation initially in English

- Need for teamwork and perseverance
- Importance of a motivated team
- Need for good planning and organising skills
- Need to be directive at times
- Knowing when to provide support
- Importance of communication and feedback
- Location and role of the facilitator influences ability to influence colleagues/change
- Impact of wider changes (e.g. management re-organisation)

During the closing meeting, the feedback was drawn together to create a visual picture that the internal facilitators felt reflected the journey they had been on during the 12 months of the project (Figure 9.2). As Figure 9.2 illustrates, the internal facilitators felt that they first had to become skilled and more confident in what they described as the 'technical' skills of facilitation, before they could tackle issues such as getting their colleagues motivated and dealing with wider contextual challenges. As their skills, knowledge and confidence developed, so too their own personal development as a facilitator began to take shape and they could see ways to apply their growing facilitation expertise within other areas of their role.

Reflections and lessons learnt

In reflecting on the experiences within this case, it is important to bear in mind that the finer details of the facilitation intervention were bound by the trial protocol. Thus although we can identify ways in which the facilitation process could be improved – or how we might do it differently if we were starting again – what was possible at the time was dictated by the overall study design. For example, reflecting on how the virtual methods of support worked, we think it would have been beneficial to include a mid-point face-to-face meeting for the facilitators to address some of the limitations of the teleconferences, for example, language difficulties and problems demonstrating how to use the audit software. Similarly, to improve continuity in the facilitation process and be prepared for possible contingencies, it would have been better to have trained two facilitators per home from the outset, rather than relying on a single facilitator who then had to identify a buddy and help get them up to speed with the details of the project. Within the FIRE study this was not possible – largely for financial reasons – but in practice we think having a pair of facilitators would have benefits, both in terms of providing cover for each other when needed, but also providing mutual support and feedback throughout the facilitation process. In some of the sites, this is how the facilitators and buddies worked together, but consistency could have been improved across all of the settings. Linked to this point, the external–internal facilitator relationship could have been strengthened further by allocating named internal facilitators to external facilitators, rather

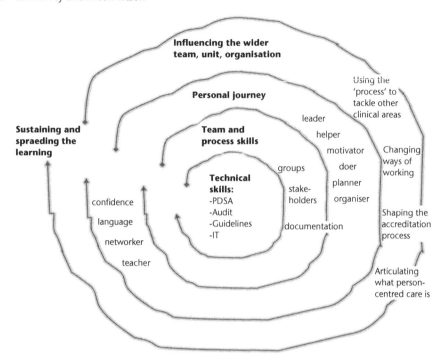

FIGURE 9.2 The internal facilitator's journey

than keeping the arrangement somewhat open. This would help in terms of encouraging ongoing communication between the internal and external facilitators outside of the formal teleconference meetings. Again in the FIRE study, this was not actively promoted because it was outside the study protocol but in the real-world setting, we believe this would be beneficial.

The experience of introducing audit was also an important learning point. Although we believe the use of data to inform and monitor improvement is valuable, in hindsight the introduction of an electronic audit system to a group of novice facilitators who had very limited face-to-face contact with each other and with the external facilitators was ambitious. This highlights a couple of important points: first, the need to simplify the audit process as far as possible; second, to weigh up the simplification of the audit process with the need for accurate data. In the FIRE experience, making the audit process more manageable for the facilitators resulted in data that did not accurately reflect the baseline. In turn, this would make it difficult to gauge the progress made at the point of re-audit. There are no easy solutions here, but our judgement is that it would have been better to undertake a full baseline audit at the start of the implementation process, rather than staging it in the way that we did. To facilitate this, we should probably have devoted more time within the initial development programme to learning about audit, reduced the number of criteria the facilitators had to collect data on and reconsidered whether PACES was a useful system to employ. In the long term, having accurate baseline data and being able to demonstrate progress and improvement over time is helpful to keep everyone engaged and informed about the project.

Linked to this point, an initial baseline audit could have been used to establish relevant and realistic goals on a home by home basis. At the residential workshop, all of the internal facilitators agreed to work towards a compliance goal of 100% for each of the audit criteria. However, as Table 9.1 illustrates, the rates of achievement varied significantly. Having an accurate baseline from which to assess current practice and then determine individualised goals may have made the project more meaningful at the nursing home level.

Another learning point that emerged relates to the availability of content expertise; this was not factored into the original design of the facilitation intervention, but was clearly an important issue for the internal facilitators. Although we were able to bring this content knowledge in via a specialist nurse, it would have been beneficial to have included it from the start of the intervention. On reflection, we would also pay more careful attention to applying the criteria for selecting facilitators. Within the FIRE study, the research team liaised with the nursing home managers to identify potential facilitators and the external facilitators had no say in who was selected for the role. However, it was clear that some of the individuals who took on the role did not meet all of the criteria, for example, in relation to their position of authority and influence within the organisation. Although it would not have directly solved the issues that arose in the FIRE study, encouraging facilitators to self-assess themselves against the criteria identified in Box 9.1 would have helped to highlight potential problems earlier on in the process. A final point relates to what happened at the end of the intervention period. In accordance with the study protocol, contact between the external and internal facilitators ceased after the 12-month intervention. In practice, this was a rather abrupt ending; in future projects, our suggestion would be to build in at least a three-month transition period to more effectively plan for the sustainability of the intervention and gradual withdrawal of the external facilitator support.

What this case study adds to our overall understanding of facilitation

At an overall study level at this point in time it is not possible to say whether the approach to facilitation described in this chapter is better than no facilitation or a more emancipatory model of facilitation. What then can we learn from participating in the process and from the formative evaluation data within the case? Our experiences suggest that it is possible to work with novice facilitators within an internal–external facilitator relationship, but that a number of key issues need to be addressed to maximise the potential of this relationship. These are as follows:

1. *Attention to the process of recruiting internal facilitators*: Although we specified explicit criteria for facilitator selection within the nursing homes, we were unable to check this out in any systematic way. Our findings reinforce how important it is to get people with the right motivation, personal confidence, credibility and level of authority in the facilitator role. More attention to checking that prospective facilitators actually meet these criteria prior to commencing in the role would be beneficial. For the approach to facilitation that we used, we would also suggest an additional criterion relating to skills and knowledge in audit and information technology.
2. *Attention to support and mentorship arrangements*: The external facilitator obviously acts as a key source of support and mentorship. However, this is often focused on the process of facilitation. It is also important to think about support requirements in relation to the content of facilitation and identifying clinical mentors who can provide specialist input and support as required. Peer support is a further consideration. From our experience, we would suggest that identifying and working with a pair of internal facilitators helps to share the work at a local level and provides much needed peer support and feedback.

3. *Attention to the internal facilitator–leader relationship*: Clear and visible support from local leaders and managers is essential for facilitators to effectively function in the role. How best to secure this local leadership support and issues relating to the formalisation of the relationship between leaders and facilitators are areas that we would suggest warrant further consideration and study.

4. *Setting realistic goals*: Alongside these strategies and actions to strengthen the internal–external facilitator approach, it is also important to recognise the amount of time that is needed to achieve the specified goals of implementing evidence into practice. In our study we allowed 12 months, which was not sufficient to reach all of the intended aims and objectives. This links to the points above about having the right people, with the right level of authority and support and the right knowledge and skills in the facilitator role. If any of these criteria are not met, it is more than likely that the implementation process will be delayed or at least slower than anticipated. Thus goals need to be established that are realistic and tailored to the local situation.

Our experience of working with the internal facilitators in the FIRE study was a valuable one and has obviously contributed to developing the model of facilitation we have presented in this book. A particularly challenging aspect of the project was providing virtual support as external facilitators to a group of internal facilitators in different countries, in different healthcare systems and, in some cases, working in a second language. This posed both logistical and contextual challenges and raised questions about whether and how virtual expert facilitation can be provided most effectively. We will reflect further on this and some of the other learning points identified in the final chapter of the book.

References

DuBeau, C., Kuchel, G., Johnson, T., Palmer, M. & Wagg, A. 2009. Committee 11. Incontinence in the frail elderly. In: Abrams, P., Cardozo, L., Khoury, S. and Wein, A. (eds) *Incontinence. 4th International Consultation on Incontinence*, pp.,961–1024 and 1796–1789. Paris: Health Publications Limited. Available: www.icsoffice.org/Publications/ICI_4/book.pdf [accessed 31 August 2014].

Harvey, G., Loftus-Hills, A., Rycroft-Malone, J., Titchen, A., Kitson, A., McCormack, B. & Seers, K. 2002. Getting evidence into practice: the role and function of facilitation. *Journal of Advanced Nursing*, 37, 577–88.

Harvey, G., Kitson, A. & Munn, Z. 2012. Promoting continence in nursing homes in four European countries: the use of PACES as a mechanism for improving the uptake of evidence-based recommendations. *International Journal of Evidence-Based Healthcare*, 10, 388–96.

Helfrich, C., Damschroder, L., Hagedorn, H., Daggett, G., Sahay, A., Ritchie, M., Damush, T., Guihan, M., Ullrich, P. & Stetler, C. 2010. A critical synthesis of literature on the promoting action on research implementation in health services (PARIHS) framework. *Implementation Science*, 5, 82.

Kitson, A., Rycroft-Malone, J., Harvey, G., McCormack, B., Seers, K. & Titchen, A. 2008. Evaluating the successful implementation of evidence into practice using the PARiHS framework: theoretical and practical challenges. *Implementation Science*, 3, 1.

Manley, K. & McCormack, B. 2003. Practice development: purpose, methodology, facilitation and evaluation. *Nursing in Critical Care*, 8, 22–9.

McCormack, B., Manley, K. & Titchen, A. 2013. *Practice Development in Nursing and Healthcare*. Chichester: John Wiley & Sons.

Seers, K., Cox, K., Crichton, N., Edwards, R., Eldh, A., Estabrooks, C., Harvey, G., Hawkes, C., Kitson, A., Linck, P., McCarthy, G., McCormack, B., Mockford, C., Rycroft-Malone, J., Titchen, A. & Wallin, L. 2012. FIRE (Facilitating Implementation of Research Evidence): a study protocol. *Implementation Science*, 7, 25.

10

USING FACILITATION TO IMPROVE NEONATAL HEALTH AND SURVIVAL IN VIETNAM

Leif Eriksson and Lars Wallin

Introduction and background to the facilitation project

This case study presents a project undertaken in Vietnam to evaluate the effectiveness of facilitation as a knowledge translation intervention for improving neonatal health and survival (Wallin et al., 2011). In terms of the facilitation intervention, key points highlighted include: implementing an external–internal model of facilitation within a large-scale research study; training laypersons to be facilitators; and undertaking implementation within a challenging context. The chapter is structured as follows. First, we present the background to the project and the reasons for choosing to study facilitation in relation to neonatal health and survival within the healthcare system of Vietnam. We then describe the facilitation model we developed for the study and outline the specific methods that were used to address the aim of improving neonatal care, to assess and manage factors relating to the local context and to engage with key stakeholders in the process of implementation. Having described the details of the intervention, we will present the research findings on the impact of the facilitation intervention. The chapter concludes with our reflections on the lessons learnt about facilitation and what we believe our study adds to the knowledge base about facilitating evidence-based healthcare.

Neonatal health and survival

The eight Millennium Development Goals were declared by the United Nations in 2000 to reduce poverty and enable sustainable development globally (United Nations General Assembly, 2000). The fourth goal aims to reduce child mortality (mortality among infants under five years of age) by two-thirds from the level in 1990 by the year 2015 (United Nations, 2006). Overall, child mortality has declined rapidly between 1990 and 2010 (UNICEF, 2012). However, mortality among infants during the first 28 days (neonatal mortality) has not decreased at the same pace (World Health Organization, 2011), meaning that the fourth Millennium Development Goal will not be reached in 2015. Worldwide, 3 million deaths occur every year during the neonatal period (Save the Children, 2013). The highest risk of dying occurs during the first 24 hours and about 75% of all neonatal deaths happen during the first week after birth (Lawn et al., 2005). There are three main causes of neonatal mortality: complications from preterm birth (35%), severe infections (23%) and birth complications (23%) (Save the Children, 2013), which all relate to suboptimal care before, during and after childbirth (Baqui et al., 2009; Lawn et al., 2009a, 2009b). To target these causes, efforts need to be focused on both women and children along a continuum of care (Kerber et al., 2007). However, the period around delivery is of particular importance (Lawn et al., 2005; Kerber et al., 2007) as 43% of the child deaths occur during the neonatal period (Save the Children, 2013).

There is a range of low-cost and evidence-based interventions that can reduce neonatal mortality by 75% if used by trained healthcare staff (Darmstadt et al., 2005; Save the Children, 2013). These interventions, such as tetanus toxoid vaccination, clean delivery practices, resuscitation of the newborn baby, breast feeding, kangaroo mother care and pneumonia management, are linked to the birth and the immediate period thereafter. It is urgent to better understand how to implement these interventions effectively (*Journal of Perinatology* Supplement, 2002), especially in low- and middle-income countries where almost all (around 98%) of the neonatal deaths occur (Save the Children, 2013).

Healthcare in Vietnam

For the past two decades, child and neonatal mortality in Vietnam have declined faster than the global average (Rajaratnam et al., 2010; Oestergaard et al., 2011; UNICEF, 2012). Trends in mortality clearly follow the political and socioeconomic climate in Vietnam, such as war, peace and different reforms (Hoa et al., 2008). However, considering that the Vietnamese government has focused on improving neonatal survival (Ministry of Health Vietnam, 2002, 2003) the reduction of neonatal mortality has still been relatively slow (Hoa et al., 2008).

In the 1980s economic reforms liberalized the health sector by introducing a number of measures such as user fees at public hospitals and expanding private medical practice (Deolalikar, 2002). The introduction of the reforms resulted in rapid economic transition in Vietnam with an accelerated period of economic growth (International Monetary Fund, 2009). In 2008, the country moved from being classified as a low-income country to a middle-income country (Cheong et al., 2010); however, the economic transition did not solely bring positive impact. For the poorest in society there were some negative consequences (Khe et al., 2002; Segall et al., 2002). For example, the high costs of healthcare resulted in poorer people seeking care less often or having to borrow money to cover their healthcare expenses (Khe et al., 2002).

The healthcare system in Vietnam has four levels (Ladinsky and Levine, 1985; Deolalikar, 2002; Dieleman et al., 2003). At the top there are national hospitals and central specialty institutes, on the second level there are provincial and regional hospitals, on the third level district hospitals and inter-communal polyclinics and on the municipality level there are commune health centres (CHCs). Primary healthcare is based around the CHCs, where staff are responsible for providing a number of healthcare programmes targeting areas such as maternal and child health, family planning, acute respiratory infections and immunization. The staffing at a CHC is typically a doctor (medical doctor or assistant doctor), a midwife and a registered nurse. In addition, village health workers (VHW) are also connected to each CHC, one for each village, providing basic healthcare for the population in their villages and being a link between the village and the healthcare system (Dieleman et al., 2003). VHWs are volunteers and they have to earn their living in other ways (Ladinsky and Levine, 1985). The VHW is particularly important when it comes to interconnecting people from ethnic minority groups with the healthcare system. In Vietnam there are 54 different ethnic groups (World Health Organization, 2003): Kinh constitute 85% of the population while the remaining 53 groups differ from Kinh in aspects such as language, social organisation, customs and other cultural systems.

Traditional medicine is integrated into the healthcare system and the Ministry of Health in Vietnam promotes the rational use of both traditional and modern therapies (Ministry of Health Vietnam, 2006). Vietnamese traditional medicine originates from both Chinese beliefs and indigenous Vietnamese practices (World Health Organization, 2001, 2002). Besides the healthcare system, there are also other stakeholders aiming to improve population health, such as the National Committee for Population, Family and Children, which provides counselling regarding family planning, and the Women's Union (www.hoilhpn.org.vn/?lang=EN), which supports women, especially those in poor and vulnerable groups.

The NeoKIP trial

The NeoKIP trial (Neonatal Knowledge Into Practice, trial registration ISRCTN44599712) was conducted in 90 communes in Quang Ninh province in Vietnam (Wallin et al., 2011). Quang Ninh is situated in the northeastern corner of Vietnam, 120 km east of the capital city Hanoi and bordering China. It is an elongated coastal province, with an area of 5900 km² having a varied geography including a large archipelago of more than 2000 islands, flat land along the coasts and mountains inland. Divided into 14 districts and 184 communes, Quang Ninh has approximately one million inhabitants belonging to more than 20 different ethnic groups; 80% are Kinh and, of the remaining groups, only five groups have a population larger than 1000. The major sources of income are tourism and coal mining.

The trial was theoretically framed by PARIHS (Promoting Action on Research Implementation in Health Services), which – as highlighted in earlier chapters – suggests that three key elements influence successful implementation of new knowledge: evidence, quality of the context in terms of coping with change, and facilitation to ensure a successful change process (Rycroft-Malone et al., 2002). We focused the research question on facilitation knowing that robust research evidence is available regarding best practice for neonatal care and that Vietnam has a relatively established and structured healthcare context. Thus, the aim of the NeoKIP cluster-randomised trial was to evaluate the effectiveness of facilitation as a knowledge translation intervention for improved neonatal health and survival (Wallin et al., 2011). The hypotheses were:

1. Interaction between healthcare practitioners and key commune members in a group supported by a facilitator and with access to evidence-based knowledge should speed up the process of practitioners changing their behaviour and subsequently improve patient outcomes.
2. Using a facilitation approach targeting local stakeholder groups should reduce the risk of neonatal deaths in the target population.

Overview of the facilitation approach

As discussed in earlier chapters, there are numerous strategies to support knowledge translation (Grol and Grimshaw, 2003), such as dissemination, education, social interaction, decision support, organisational and patient-oriented strategies (Wallin, 2009). Despite considerable research effort there is still uncertainty about how and when specific strategies should be used to obtain the best results (Bero et al., 1998; Grol and Grimshaw, 2003; Thompson et al., 2007). However, strategies that have social interaction as a major component appear promising (Nilsen et al., 2010), such as using a change agent, linking agent, facilitator, champion, knowledge broker, opinion leader or educational outreach (Thompson et al., 2006). Some of these strategies depend upon a person with expert knowledge on the topic interacting with individuals or groups in order to influence and change practice. This is not typically the case with facilitation where the facilitator's input is primarily focused around their interpersonal and group management skills, as opposed to expertise in the implementation topic (Harvey et al., 2002; Wallin et al., 2005a; Stetler et al., 2006; Dogherty et al., 2010).

Most studies on facilitation as a knowledge translation method have been performed in high-income countries (Harvey et al., 2002; Ellis et al., 2005; Wallin et al., 2005a, 2005b; Stetler et al., 2006; Thompson et al., 2006; Dogherty et al., 2010, 2012). However, during the last 5–10 years, studies in low- and middle-income countries have increasingly focused on community mobilisation through different bottom-up approaches, among them some studies evaluating the use of facilitation (Rosato et al., 2008; Nair et al., 2010; Lassi and Bhutta, 2011). A project in Bolivia, where efforts in strengthening women's groups succeeded in lowering perinatal mortality by more than 60% (O'Rourke et al., 1998), influenced many subsequent and successful projects focusing on community-based strategies in South Asia (Bang et al., 2005; Jokhio et al., 2005; Baqui et al., 2008; Kumar et al., 2008; Bhutta et al., 2011). For example, in Nepal, a project using facilitators to target women's groups resulted in a 30% reduction in neonatal mortality, with a corresponding increase in uptake of antenatal care, more institutional deliveries, skilled birth attendance and improvements in hygiene aspects of care (Manandhar et al., 2004; Morrison et al., 2005). Studies in India (Tripathy et al., 2010) and Bangladesh (Azad et al., 2010) using a similar design as in the Nepal study were successful in improving healthcare practices and changing behaviour in the intervention sites. The Indian study showed a reduction of neonatal mortality comparable to that seen in Nepal, while the study in Bangladesh, which was a scale-up attempt of the intervention, failed to show any impact on newborn survival. A meta-analysis, including the trials mentioned above, showed significantly reduced neonatal mortality with facilitated women's group interventions if the population coverage was 450–750 per group (Prost et al., 2013). In the Bangladesh study each group covered a population of more than 1400 (Azad et al., 2010). When designing the NeoKIP trial we aimed to have an intervention that could be scaled up and have sustainable effects. Therefore, in the NeoKIP intervention we chose to target groups that were parts of the healthcare system and used facilitators who belonged to established organisations in Vietnamese society.

Based on data from a baseline survey, districts in Quang Ninh having a neonatal mortality rate ≥15 deaths per 1000 live births (15/1000) were included in the trial (Wallin et al., 2011). Hence, eight districts with a total of 90 communes were included; 44 communes were randomly allocated as intervention sites and 46 as control sites (Figure 10.1). The study area housed approximately 350 000 inhabitants and the overall neonatal mortality rate was 24/1000.

After a pilot we decided to recruit NeoKIP facilitators from the Women's Union, a nationwide organisation established in the 1930s. The Women's Union has a long tradition

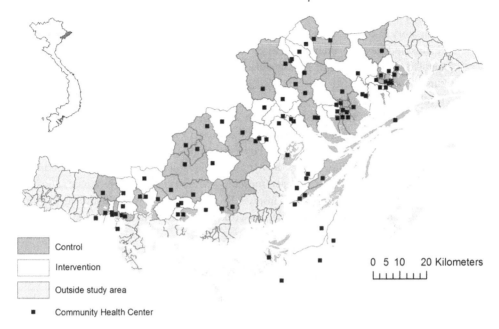

FIGURE 10.1 Study area with intervention and control communes in Quang Ninh province, Vietnam

of involvement at local and regional levels, particularly in healthcare matters. However, in relation to healthcare they were viewed as laypersons. It has previously been recognised that a facilitator can be either internal or external to the group that is targeted (Harvey et al., 2002; Stetler et al., 2006; Dogherty et al., 2010). In the NeoKIP intervention, the facilitators were geographically internal (i.e. they came from the same part of the province that they later worked in as a facilitator), but external with regard to the team at the CHC, the topic area (newborn healthcare) and the fact that they were not healthcare professionals. The rationale for using facilitators from the Women's Union was primarily the increased potential for sustainability and scale-up. Selecting one of the healthcare workers at each CHC as a facilitator was an alternative strategy. However, supporting 44 instead of 8 facilitators over three years would have been a difficult task in terms of providing and evaluating a homogenous intervention of high quality. We also anticipated that using healthcare professionals as facilitators could have limited the groups to focus primarily on problems and actions linked to the immediate healthcare service.

The NeoKIP facilitators were trained for two weeks in group dynamics, basic evidence-based neonatal care (Ministry of Health Vietnam, 2002) and quality improvement methods, such as the Plan–Do–Study–Act (PDSA) cycle (Langley et al., 2009) to prepare them to facilitate the work in the 44 intervention sites.

In each of the 44 intervention sites, a maternal and newborn health group (MNHG) was established as the focus for implementation activity (these groups are described in more detail later in the chapter). In order to cover eight facilitator positions for 44 MNHGs during the three intervention years, 11 facilitators were recruited and trained at two separate occasions (8 before the start of the intervention and 3 half-way though the intervention period due to withdrawals). During the intervention all facilitators met jointly with supervisors (external facilitators from the Vietnamese research team) once a month, for two consecutive days, to discuss and develop their facilitation roles. The supervisors also attended MNHG meetings regularly to observe and give feedback to the facilitator in charge. In addition, facilitators supervised each other (i.e. attended meetings facilitated by colleagues to observe and give feedback on performance).

The facilitators were also trained to encourage the MNHG members to use the National Guidelines in Reproductive Health Care (Ministry of Health Vietnam, 2002) when identifying problems and formulating actions. These evidence-based guidelines were introduced in 2003 in line with a campaign run by the Ministry of Health in Vietnam focused on improving peri-natal health and lowering neonatal mortality (Ministry of Health Vietnam, 2003). The way of working in this intervention was inspired by others evaluating facilitation as an implementation support intervention, for example the work by Rycroft-Malone and colleagues in the POISE trial (Rycroft-Malone et al., 2012).

Implementing the evidence: project design

In order to assess the situation prior to the start of the implementation period, a baseline study was conducted in all 14 districts of Quang Ninh province in 2006, primarily collecting data concerning the number of live births and neonatal deaths for 2005 (Wallin et al., 2011). Addi-tionally, both quantitative and qualitative data were gathered to examine the conditions for neonates, their families and the primary healthcare system. A number of studies conducted dur-ing the baseline survey in Quang Ninh indicated several challenges regarding neonatal health. In 2005 the neonatal mortality rate in our baseline survey was found to be 16/1000, although official statistics reported a neonatal mortality rate of 4/1000, raising a concern about under-reporting (Målqvist et al., 2008a). Furthermore, the 14 districts in Quang Ninh demonstrated a range in neonatal mortality rates from 10 to 44/1000. The high-mortality districts were situated in rural and mountainous areas with mortality rates similar to those of low-income countries, while urban areas had mortality rates similar to those of high-income countries (UNICEF, 2012; World Bank, 2012). Moreover, neonates of mothers having a long distance to travel to a health facility (CHC or hospital) and belonging to an ethnic minority group had a strikingly increased risk of dying during the neonatal period (Målqvist et al., 2010, 2011). We also found that many of the neonatal death cases never had any contact with the healthcare system (Målqvist et al., 2008b) and that there was a strong correlation between neonatal death and home deliveries (Nga et al., 2010). The results from the baseline survey demonstrated a severe situation for the neonates and their families and significant potential for improvement if effective and inexpensive interventions were implemented.

Methods used to assess and respond to contextual issues

During the baseline survey 412 primary healthcare staff (physicians, midwives and registered nurses) responded to a knowledge survey regarding basic and evidence-based procedures in neonatal care (Eriksson et al., 2009). The knowledge survey was conducted in 12 of the 14 districts. Overall, the survey participants achieved 60% of the maximal score. Based on the total score of the survey in each district, the six districts with the highest mean scores and the six districts with the lowest mean scores formed two distinct geographical areas (the northeast districts and the southwest districts). Besides differing in the level of staff knowledge, the two geographical areas also differed with regards to other parameters related to neonatal health. In the northeast districts the neonatal mortality rate was 50% higher, the number of pregnant women attending antenatal care three times or more was 35% lower, the accessibility of evidence-based guidelines 20% lower and the distance from the CHCs to any of the tertiary hospitals was, on average, three times longer than in the southwest districts. Hence, a newborn child in the northeast districts was not only cared for by staff with a lower level of basic knowledge, it also had a higher risk of dying during the first four weeks after delivery and, if it became seriously ill, had a longer distance to travel to a tertiary hospital than a newborn child in the southwest districts. It is well known that ethnic minority groups in Vietnam are more disadvantaged than the Kinh population, for example, in terms of education and health (World Health Organization, 2003; Målqvist et al., 2011). The findings from the knowledge survey verify these differences as the northeast districts had a larger proportion of ethnic minorities than the southwest districts. Hence, the inequalities between the two geographical areas suggest that all children did not have the same basic opportunity to become healthy and even survive.

As a follow-up to the baseline knowledge survey, focus group discussions were conducted with primary healthcare staff (mainly physicians and midwives) aiming to explore how knowledge translation was performed in primary healthcare settings in the province, which helped us to identify potential barriers to the implementation of evidence-based practice (Eriksson et al., 2011). Focus group participants described several channels for acquisition and management of knowledge. For example, training was perceived as the best way to acquire knowledge and a necessity for providing good service at the CHCs. The perinatal guidelines from 2003 (Ministry of Health Vietnam, 2002) were perceived as a relevant source of information. However, it was claimed that the guidelines were rarely used, mainly because of their poor introduction and the competition from other written material. Furthermore, primary healthcare staff asked for more interaction with colleagues at higher levels in the healthcare system. Staff knowledge and skills were perceived as scarce, with negative consequences for the healthcare system and patient care. Traditional medicine, a relatively low number of deliveries, low availability of equipment and drugs, CHCs located in rural or mountainous locations and poorly paid staff were identified as barriers to a well-functioning healthcare context and improvement of staff skills (see Box 10.1 for examples of barriers).

BOX 10.1   PERCEIVED BARRIERS TO THE IMPLEMENTATION OF EVIDENCE-BASED CARE

The low number of deliveries at the CHCs influenced the level of knowledge and skills among staff. In the study province, two-thirds of the CHCs assisted fewer than 18 deliveries each in 2005 (Nga et al., 2010). This low activity is largely a result of the health sector reforms in the 1980s (Witter, 1996), which influenced the population to seek care in the private healthcare sector and at the higher levels of the governmental healthcare system (Deolalikar, 2002; Ngo and Hill, 2011). Thus, the primary healthcare level experienced a reduction in clinical activity, for example, of assisted deliveries, which implies a risk of reduced quality of care (Scotland and Bullough, 2004).

(continued)

(continued)

Lack of resources and poor salaries impeded the development of enhanced staff knowledge and skills. In Vietnam it has been shown that physicians prefer to work at hospitals rather than at the primary healthcare level because of better salaries, more resources and better working conditions (Witter et al., 2011). Furthermore, in northern Vietnam, healthcare staff at the primary healthcare level identified low income as the most discouraging factor in their work (Dieleman et al., 2003). The VHWs in Vietnam might lack motivation to perform well, despite being an important bridge between the population and the healthcare system as they have a relatively low monthly income. The VHW positions are most important in rural and mountainous areas (Ladinsky and Levine, 1985; Ngo and Hill, 2011), which implies that the most disadvantaged groups in society, those belonging to ethnic minorities, are dependent on the low-paid and therefore potentially less committed VHWs. In a recent study, healthcare providers and patients perceived the use of CHCs to be a cost-effective strategy, with the potential to reach the whole population with regard to reproductive healthcare (Ngo and Hill, 2011). However, they also perceived the current standard of the CHCs to be too low, especially in rural and mountainous areas where the CHCs have a central function because of the long distance to hospitals.

Although National Guidelines in Reproductive Health Care were available, (Ministry of Health Vietnam, 2002) they were not frequently used by primary healthcare staff, although they were implemented as tools at the CHCs for staff to perform reproductive health care. Reasons for this low level of use can be attributed to poor introduction of the guidelines, the existence of other written material and competition with traditional medicine. In general, primary healthcare staff used evidence based on patient and clinical experiences.

The underreporting of neonatal deaths in the study province (Målqvist et al., 2008a) could be indicative of the culture not valuing local data as important and therefore not a priority for the CHC staff. Such underreporting could also result in poor decisions being made in relation to the planning of care and resource allocation.

From this baseline analysis, it is clear that a number of contextual factors were present that created a potential challenge in relation to implementation. The geographical setting of the study and the distinct variation between different geographical locations was an important consideration, along with issues relating to the workforce knowledge, skills, support and motivation. Furthermore, the PARIHS framework suggests that receptiveness to change is greater in a rich context (Rycroft-Malone et al., 2002). Such a context should exhibit decentralised decision-making (Rycroft-Malone, 2004), with an emphasis on a respectful collaboration between managers and workers and where the management style is facilitative rather than directive. However, during the time of the baseline study, this kind of context did not exist in Quang Ninh. Rather the Vietnamese healthcare system is hierarchically structured (Ladinsky and Levine, 1985; Dieleman et al., 2003) and known to perform knowledge translation in a top-down manner (Laverack and Tuan, 2001). Most likely, this way of working is influenced by Confucianism, which is a dominant philosophy in Vietnam, placing a strong emphasis on hierarchy (Hägerdal, 2005).

From the NeoKIP baseline survey we learned that many difficult contextual conditions existed in the study province. To be able to attend to these circumstances through an intervention we believed that it was important to recruit local facilitators who would be familiar with the context and to allow the intervention groups to decide on the problems and actions that they wanted to work with. To test the knowledge translation intervention of the NeoKIP trial, which can be characterized as a bottom-up and interactive approach tailored to fit the local context (Wallin et al., 2011), was both challenging and interesting in a top-down health system.

Methods used to identify and work with stakeholders

As described, a maternal and newborn health group (MNHG) was set up in each of the 44 intervention communes, adhering to a directive from the provincial health bureau. This group typically consisted of eight participants: the vice chairperson of the commune (having responsibility for health in the commune), three primary healthcare staff (typically a doctor, a midwife and a registered nurse), a VHW, two representatives from the Women's Union (the chair at the commune level and a member at the village level) and a population motivator from the National Committee for Population, Family and Children. We felt that having a mix of influential individuals working to improve newborn health would increase the understanding of the local health situation and the opportunity to reach out to and influence different levels in society.

The overall intention was that the facilitators should enable and support MNHG members who had both local and practical knowledge to improve neonatal health and survival in the area. Each MNHG met monthly with a facilitator for 2–3 hours. The PDSA cycle was the basic structure for the MNHGs' work: cycles were used to identify and prioritise local problem(s) and actions (Plan), implement the actions (Do), evaluate the implementation process by using process indicators for the targeted problem(s) (Study), and then reconsider the problem-solving strategy (Act) (Figure 10.2). Hence, in each intervention commune the MNHGs were free to prioritise problems and implement actions according to needs and feasibility.

Evaluating the impact of facilitation

At each meeting with an MNHG, the facilitator filled in a diary where she summarised the meeting in her own words and entered data on meeting time, attendance, what problems and actions the MNHGs identified and prioritised. The rationale for the diaries was both to collect data on the process and to help the MNHGs in their work. During the intervention period comprehensive data collection was carried out on neonatal deaths, live births, healthcare parameters and the intervention process.

Of the 44 MNHGs, 43 were active until the end of the intervention period. Only one MNHG withdrew from the NeoKIP trial, and this was after 21 months (i.e. 15 months before the end of the trial). In total, the MNHGs conducted 95% (1508/1584) of the intended monthly meetings and the overall attendance of the MNHG members was 86%.

The members in the 44 MNHGs identified 32 types of problem that were addressed 206 times and implemented 39 types of actions that were applied 933 times over the three intervention years (Box 10.2). Actions taken to target the problems were mainly based on applying different communication approaches.

Plan

Identify local problems
and plan actions

Do

Implement action

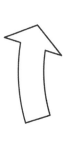

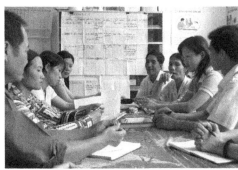

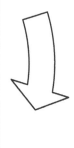

Act

Reconsider the
strategy

Study

Evaluate results

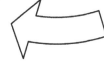

FIGURE 10.2 A Plan–Do–Study–Act cycle in maternal and newborn health group. Photo: Daniel
Persson

**BOX 10.2 MOST FREQUENTLY REPORTED PROBLEMS AND
ACTIONS**

Most frequently identified problems:

- Low frequency of antenatal care visits (42 times)
- Low frequency of postnatal home visits (33)
- Low awareness among pregnant women of the importance of diet, work and rest
  (23)
- High frequency of home deliveries (16)
- Low awareness of breastfeeding practices (14)

Most frequently used actions:

- Communication activities (623 times)[a]
- Preparation of educational material and training of Village Health Workers (154)
- Postnatal home visits (63)
- Creation of lists of pregnant and newly delivered women (28)
- Distribution of leaflets (25)

[a]These included a range of activities that aimed to mobilise or counsel women at home, communicate messages at meetings, counsel women at CHCs, communicate messages through loudspeakers, etc.

The third year of the intervention resulted in a reduced neonatal mortality of 49% [adjusted odds ratio (OR_{adj}) 0.51; 95% confidence interval (CI) 0.30–0.89] after a latent period and the 44 intervention communes had a longitudinally downward trend (Persson et al., 2013). In detail, the neonatal mortality rate of the 22 377 live births from July 2008 to June 2011 was 19.1, 19.0 and 11.6/1000 live births in the intervention communes and 23.9, 18.0 and 21.1 in the control communes during the three years (Figure 10.3).

Data from a random sample of mothers with live births (n = 1243) showed that women in intervention communes had a higher attendance at antenatal care than women in control communes (OR 2.27, 95% CI 1.07–4.80). This result concurred with process data showing low attendance at antenatal care as the top priority problem. However, when investigating another top priority problem – postnatal home visits – no difference was detected between women in intervention and control communes (Persson et al., 2013).

Qualitative data were collected in 15 focus group discussions with facilitators (n = 3) and a sample of MNHGs (n = 12) at different time points to study the facilitation process and

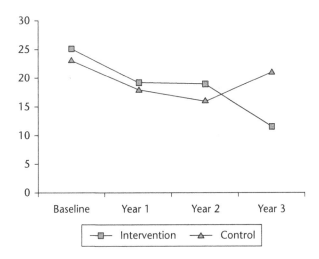

FIGURE 10.3 Neonatal mortality rates for intervention and control communes

identified barriers (Eriksson et al., 2013). Facilitators and MNHG members agreed during the discussions that having intervention groups representing various organisations was beneficial for them as stakeholders and for neonatal health in the communes. The MNHG members commented on the fact that they met regularly and that all members were active and contributed to discussions and actions, but often with the chair of the group acting as the main decision-maker. The behaviour of the chair of the group influenced other group members' behaviour; for example, if a chair was interested and engaged the other group members became engaged in their group's work, while an unfocused chair influenced group members negatively. The facilitators experienced that they were more successful when they invested time before and during the intervention to establish and maintain a good relationship with the chair of the group. Furthermore, to function well as a facilitator required effort in adapting to the local context.

At one level, the MNHGs in the NeoKIP trial could be viewed as community coalitions (i.e. groups of people having a joint venture to make change and introduce innovative solutions to health problems) (Butterfoss, 2006). However, a key feature of a community coalition is an agreement to work together, which does not necessarily apply in the current study as the groups were established by the NeoKIP researchers in collaboration with local authorities. Consequently, the sense of local ownership was probably not that strong, at least at the outset, which might have resulted in a lack of motivation among MNHG members to engage in the project (Eriksson et al., 2013). Despite these conditions the facilitators persistently continued with their task to support the MNHGs in their work in identifying problems and implementing actions. In the NeoKIP intervention the facilitators faced both negative and positive attitudes and behaviours when meeting the MNHGs. In particular, the MNHG members were critical about being supported by facilitators lacking clinical knowledge. However, overall the MNHG members' engagement and enthusiasm increased over time. A common perceived problem with the NeoKIP intervention was the lack of financial support to the MNHGs. Contrary to the research perspective, that the work in the MNHG should be viewed as ordinary work, MNHG members perceived that reimbursement was necessary to motivate them to meet monthly targets and to implement actions in the communes. They also expressed a view that the lack of resources acted as a restraint to implementing the proposed actions and interaction with the population.

Reflections and lessons learnt

It was two years before differences in neonatal mortality between intervention and control communes were detected. For the effect to occur after a latent period was to some extent expected as we were evaluating a complex social intervention (Persson et al., 2013). Several factors might have contributed to the delayed effect, such as the need for time for the MNHGs to function properly and for facilitators to develop the necessary skills and acclimatise themselves within the various communes. In the following sections we will discuss some aspects of the facilitator role and how it worked within the NeoKIP trial.

A number of characteristics for facilitators of change have been suggested to be important for community mobilisation projects aimed at improving maternal, newborn and child health (Rosato et al., 2008) (Box 10.3).

BOX 10.3   IMPORTANT CHARACTERISTICS FOR FACILITATORS OF CHANGE IN COMMUNITY MOBILISATION

- Credibility in the commune
- Knowledge of community structures and protocols
- Cultural sensitivity
- Interpersonal communication skills
- Interest in being a facilitator
- Interest in maternal and newborn health
- Language skills
- Affiliation with and support from an organisation
- Time to do the work

Through the process evaluation of the NeoKIP intervention we realised that the facilitators did not fulfil all these criteria. The facilitators expressed a view that to become a successful facilitator required a range of skills and extensive commitment. They also felt that they received inadequate support to effectively carry out their role; the training was considered too short and complicated and they did not experience sufficient support from either the research team or the organisations involved throughout the intervention. Both facilitators and MNHG members initially considered their lack of health knowledge as a barrier and their confidence in acting as facilitators was low. MNHG members had expected to be assisted by someone with superior knowledge. These expectations influenced some of the MNHG members to see the facilitator as an unnecessary person who did not provide any significant support. This, however, changed over time and both parties thought that facilitators' performance and skills increased over the intervention period.

The choice of using laypersons as facilitators was controversial and was criticised both by the facilitators themselves and the MNHG members. Harvey et al. (2002) suggest that a facilitator should have a blend of personal attributes and management skills to achieve effective facilitation, while Stetler et al. (2006) suggest that it is critical that facilitators have knowledge on evidence-based practice. Despite the limited knowledge on the topic areas among the facilitators in the NeoKIP trail and the associated problems they faced, we still think that recruiting laypersons was the best option, primarily because of the ability to implement a cost-effective intervention with real opportunities to scale-up. It is also important to bear in mind that successful facilitation is a team effort (Dogherty et al., 2010, 2012). In NeoKIP the facilitator–MNHG teams succeeded in changing attitudes and behaviour among healthcare staff and pregnant women in the intervention communes, which led to improved neonatal survival. This success needs to be considered as a joint achievement of facilitators and MNHG members. However, a lesson learned from this project was not to underestimate the time needed for preparing facilitators and MNHGs (i.e. to have somewhat longer training to ensure that facilitators felt better prepared and make sure that all MNHGs were informed about the requirements of being involved in the intervention).

To succeed as a facilitator it was essential to have a good relationship with the chair of the MNHG. It has been described that having a group leader is a key prerequisite for the function of a successful group coalition (O'Neill et al., 1997; Stetler et al., 2006; Dogherty et al., 2010, 2012). In the NeoKIP trial, when facilitators and the chair of the MNHG established a good relationship, the other MNHG members performed better and the facilitators' credibility in both the MNHGs and in the communes was enhanced. For the MNHG members it was a new experience to work with a facilitator. They described that the facilitators engaged in meetings and activities in an enthusiastic way. However, when the facilitators changed frequently or when they were unfamiliar with the cultural context of a particular commune, they were described as barriers for the MNHG in implementing their actions. Hence, it was important for facilitators to know and adapt to the local culture.

Although the NeoKIP intervention was successful in reducing neonatal mortality we believe the intervention has great potential for improvement; in turn this could help to improve neonatal survival to an even greater extent, particularly if applied in areas with high levels of neonatal mortality. Furthermore, because it is cost-effective, the NeoKIP intervention has potential to change existing patterns of high neonatal mortality rates in many low-income countries. The total incremental cost per birthing woman in the NeoKIP intervention was calculated to be US$6.5 (Persson et al., 2013), which must be considered a low cost for such a comprehensive intervention.

What this case study adds to our understanding of facilitation?

In the NeoKIP trial we demonstrated that local stakeholder groups composed of primary care staff and local politicians supported by a facilitator working with a problem-solving approach improved healthcare practices and reduced neonatal mortality over a three-year period. A process evaluation of this intervention showed that having members in the intervention groups representing various organisations and with influential positions in the commune was beneficial. Furthermore, it was possible to train laypersons to act as facilitators and they functioned best with the groups when they established a good relationship with the chairs of the group and were familiar with the local context. The evaluation further indicated that the PDSA cycle was a very useful tool in assisting stakeholders to structure their work. Although Vietnam has a hierarchical healthcare context, it was possible to implement this bottom-up approach and accomplish remarkable results. Despite these promising results we can also see that there is plenty of room for improving the facilitation approach we used in the NeoKIP study.

At the time of writing, three years after ending the NeoKIP trial, our research team has received funding for continuation of the studies in Vietnam. As a first step we will conduct a follow-up survey in the Quang Ninh province to see if the reduction in neonatal mortality rates has been sustained after ending the trial. We will also go back to the intervention communes where we held focus group interviews with MNHG members to ask if they have continued the work in any way and how they retrospectively look upon the achievements that were made during the intervention period. Additionally we will interview community leaders on what impact the work and results of the NeoKIP intervention has generated in terms of policy changes and/or activities in the communes.

Because of the promising outcomes of the NeoKIP trail we are also aiming for a scaled-up study in six poor provinces in northern Vietnam with higher neonatal mortality rates than in Quang Ninh. In that study we will add to the community approach through a facilitation intervention in district hospitals with a focus on the departments where delivering women and newborns are cared for. In the hospitals we will, however, recruit and train healthcare professionals for the facilitator role instead of laypersons. We believe these two planned studies will generate interesting results on the long-term sustainability of a knowledge translation intervention as well as the effects and experience of scaling-up the facilitation intervention in more disadvantaged populations.

References

Azad, K., Barnett, S., Banerjee, B., Shaha, S., Khan, K., Rego, A.R., Barua, S., Flatman, D., et al. 2010. Effect of scaling up women's groups on birth outcomes in three rural districts in Bangladesh: a cluster-randomised controlled trial. *Lancet*, 375, 1193–202.

Bang, A.T., Bang, R.A. & Reddy, H.M. 2005. Home-based neonatal care: summary and applications of the field trial in rural Gadchiroli, India (1993 to 2003). *Journal of Perinatology*, 25(Suppl 1), S108–22.

Baqui, A.H., El-Arifeen, S., Darmstadt, G.L., Ahmed, S., Williams, E.K., Seraji, H.R., et al. 2008. Effect of community-based newborn-care intervention package implemented through two service-delivery strategies in Sylhet district, Bangladesh: a cluster-randomised controlled trial. *Lancet*, 371, 1936–44.

Baqui, A.H., Ahmed, S., El Arifeen, S., Darmstadt, G.L., Rosecrans, A.M., Mannan, I., et al. 2009. Effect of timing of first postnatal care home visit on neonatal mortality in Bangladesh: a observational cohort study. *British Medical Journal*, 339, b2826.

Bero, L.A., Grilli, R., Grimshaw, J.M., Harvey, E., Oxman, A.D. & Thomson, M.A. 1998. Closing the gap between research and practice: an overview of systematic reviews of interventions to promote the implementation of research findings. The Cochrane Effective Practice and Organization of Care Review Group. *British Medical Journal*, 317, 465–8.

Bhutta, Z.A., Soofi, S., Cousens, S., Mohammad, S., Memon, Z.A., Ali, I., et al. 2011. Improvement of perinatal and newborn care in rural Pakistan through community-based strategies: a cluster-randomised effectiveness trial. *Lancet*, 377, 403–12.

Butterfoss, F.D. 2006. Process evaluation for community participation. *Annual Review of Public Health*, 27, 323–40.

Cheong, K.-C., Duc, P.M. & Thang, N. (eds) 2010. *From Low-Income to Industrialized: Vietnam in the Next Decade and Beyond*. Hanoi: Vietnam Academy of Social Sciences/World Bank.

Darmstadt, G.L., Bhutta, Z.A., Cousens, S., Adam, T., Walker, N. & De Bernis, L. 2005. Evidence-based, cost-effective interventions: how many newborn babies can we save? *Lancet*, 365, 977–88.

Deolalikar, A.B. 2002. Access to health services by the poor and the non-poor: the case of Vietnam. *Journal of Asian and African Studies*, 37, 244–61.

Dieleman, M., Cuong, P.V., Anh, L.V. & Martineau, T. 2003. Identifying factors for job motivation of rural health workers in North Viet Nam. *Human Resources for Health*, 1, 10.

Dogherty, E.J., Harrison, M.B. & Graham, I.D. 2010. Facilitation as a role and process in achieving evidence-based practice in nursing: a focused review of concept and meaning. *Worldviews on Evidence Based Nursing*, 7, 76–89.

Dogherty, E.J., Harrison, M.B., Baker, C. & Graham, I.D. 2012. Following a natural experiment of guideline adaptation and early implementation: a mixed-methods study of facilitation. *Implementation Science*, 7, 9.

Ellis, I., Howard, P., Larson, A. & Robertson, J. 2005. From workshop to work practice: an exploration of context and facilitation in the development of evidence-based practice. *Worldviews on Evidence Based Nursing*, 2, 84–93.

Eriksson, L., Nga, N.T., Målqvist, M., Persson, L.Å., Ewald, U. & Wallin, L. 2009. Evidence-based practice in neonatal health: knowledge among primary health care staff in northern Vietnam. *Human Resources for Health*, 7, 36.

Eriksson, L., Nga, N.T., Hoa, D.P., Persson, L.A., Ewald, U. & Wallin, L. 2011. Newborn care and knowledge translation – perceptions among primary health care staff in northern Vietnam. *Implementation Science*, 6, 29.

Eriksson, L., Duc, D.M., Eldh, A.C., Vu, P.N., Tran, Q.H., Målqvist, M. & Wallin, L. 2013. Lessons learned from stakeholders in a facilitation intervention targeting neonatal health in Quang Ninh province, Vietnam. *BMC Pregnancy and Childbirth*, 13, 234.

Grol, R. & Grimshaw, J. 2003. From best evidence to best practice: effective implementation of change in patients' care. *Lancet*, 362, 1225–30.

Hägerdal, H. 2005. *Vietnams historia*. Lund: Historiska Media.

Harvey, G., Loftus-Hills, A., Rycroft-Malone, J., Titchen, A., Kitson, A., McCormack, B. & Seers, K. 2002. Getting evidence into practice: the role and function of facilitation. *Journal of Advanced Nursing*, 37, 577–88.

Hoa, D.P., Nga, N.T., Malqvist, M. & Persson, L.A. 2008. Persistent neonatal mortality despite improved under-five survival: a retrospective cohort study in northern Vietnam. *Acta Paediatrica*, 97, 166–70.

International Monetary Fund 2009. *World Economic Outlook, April 2009: Crisis and Recovery*. Washington, DC: International Monetary Fund.

Jokhio, A.H., Winter, H.R. & Cheng, K.K. 2005. An intervention involving traditional birth attendants and perinatal and maternal mortality in Pakistan. *New England Journal of Medicine*, 352, 2091–9.

Journal of Perinatology Supplement 2002. Executive summary. *Journal of Perinatology*, 3–4.

Kerber, K.J., De Graft-Johnson, J.E., Bhutta, Z.A., Okong, P., Starrs, A. & Lawn, J.E. 2007. Continuum of care for maternal, newborn, and child health: from slogan to service delivery. *Lancet*, 370, 1358–69.

Khe, N.D., Toan, N.V., Xuan, L.T., Eriksson, B., Hojer, B. & Diwan, V.K. 2002. Primary health concept revisited: where do people seek health care in a rural area of Vietnam? *Health Policy*, 61, 95–109.

Kumar, V., Mohanty, S., Kumar, A., Misra, R.P., Santosham, M., Awasthi, S., et al. 2008. Effect of community-based behaviour change management on neonatal mortality in Shivgarh, Uttar Pradesh, India: a cluster-randomised controlled trial. *Lancet*, 372, 1151–62.

Ladinsky, J.L. & Levine, R.E. 1985. The organization of health services in Vietnam. *Journal of Public Health Policy*, 6, 255–68.

Langley, G., Moen, R., Nolan, K., Nolan, T., Norman, C & Provost, L. 2009. *The Improvement Guide. A Practical Approach to Enhancing Organizational Performance. 2nd edition*. Chichester: Jossey Bass Wiley.

Lassi, Z.S. & Bhutta, Z.A. 2011. Unfolding the universe of newborn health interventions: the role of innovative community-based strategies. BJOG: An *International Journal of Obstetrics and Gynaecology*, 118(Suppl 2), 18–21.

Laverack, G. & Tuan, T. 2001. *Effective Information, Education and Communication in Vietnam*. Hanoi: UNICEF.

Lawn, J.E., Cousens, S. & Zupan, J. 2005. 4 million neonatal deaths: When? Where? Why? *Lancet*, 365, 891–900.

Lawn, J.E., Kerber, K., Enweronu-Laryea, C. & Massee Bateman, O. 2009a. Newborn survival in low resource settings – are we delivering? *International Journal of Obstetrics and Gynaecology*, 116(Suppl 1), 49–59.

Lawn, J.E., Lee, A.C., Kinney, M., Sibley, L., Carlo, W.A., Paul, V.K., Pattinson, R. & Darmstadt, G.L. 2009b. Two million intrapartum-related stillbirths and neonatal deaths: where, why, and what can be done? *International Journal of Gynecology and Obstetrics*, 107(Suppl 1), S5–18, S19.

Målqvist, M., Eriksson, L., Nga, N.T., Fagerland, L.I., Hoa, D.P., Wallin, L., Ewald, U. & Persson, L.A. 2008a. Unreported births and deaths, a severe obstacle for improved neonatal survival in low-income countries; a population based study. *BMC International Health and Human Rights*, 8, 4.

Målqvist, M., Nga, N.T., Eriksson, L., Wallin, L., Ewald, U. & Persson, L.A. 2008b. Delivery care utilisation and care-seeking in the neonatal period: a population-based study in Vietnam. *Annals of Tropical Paediatrics*, 28, 191–8.Målqvist, M., Sohel, N., Do, T.T., Eriksson, L. & Persson, L.A. 2010. Distance decay in delivery care utilisation associated with neonatal mortality. A case referent study in northern Vietnam. *BMC Public Health*, 10, 762.

Målqvist, M., Nga, N.T., Eriksson, L., Wallin, L., Hoa, D.P. & Persson, L.A. 2011. Ethnic inequity in neonatal survival: a case-referent study in northern Vietnam. *Acta Paediatrica*, 100, 340–6.

Manandhar, D.S., Osrin, D., Shrestha, B.P., Mesko, N., Morrison, J., Tumbahangphe, K.M., et al. 2004. Effect of a participatory intervention with women's groups on birth outcomes in Nepal: cluster-randomised controlled trial. *Lancet*, 364, 970–9.

Ministry of Health Vietnam 2002. *National Standards and Guidelines for Reproductive Health Care Services.* Hanoi: Ministry of Health.

Ministry of Health Vietnam 2003. *Ministry of Health Directive on Newborn Health: 04/2003/CT-BYT.* Hanoi: Ministry of Health.

Ministry of Health Vietnam 2006. *Comprehensive Development Design for the Health System in Viet Nam to 2010 and Vision by 2020.* Hanoi: Ministry of Health.

Morrison, J., Tamang, S., Mesko, N., Osrin, D., Shrestha, B., Manandhar, M., et al. 2005. Women's health groups to improve perinatal care in rural Nepal. *BMC Pregnancy and Childbirth*, 5, 6.

Nair, N., Tripathy, P., Prost, A., Costello, A. & Osrin, D. 2010. Improving newborn survival in low-income countries: community-based approaches and lessons from South Asia. *PLoS Medicine*, 7, e1000246.

Nga, N.T., Målqvist, M., Eriksson, L., Hoa, D.P., Johansson, A., Wallin, L., Persson, L.A. & Ewald, U. 2010. Perinatal services and outcomes in Quang Ninh province, Vietnam. *Acta Paediatrica*, 99, 1478–83.

Ngo, A.D. & Hill, P.S. 2011. Quality of reproductive health services at commune health stations in Viet Nam: implications for national reproductive health care strategy. *Reproductive Health Matters*, 19, 52–61.

Nilsen, P., Roback, K. & Krevers, B. 2010. Förklaringsfaktorer för implementeringsutfall – ett ramverk. In: Nilsen, P. (ed.) *Implementering. Teori och tillämpning inom hälso-& sjukvård.* Lund: Studentlitteratur AB.

O'Neill, M., Lemieux, V., Groleau, G., Fortin, J.-P.A. & Lamarche, P. 1997. Coalition theory as a framework for understanding and implementing intersectoral health-related interventions. *Health Promotion International*, 12, 79–87.

O'Rourke, K., Howard-Grabman, L. & Seoane, G. 1998. Impact of community organization of women on perinatal outcomes in rural Bolivia. *The Revista Panamericana de Salud Pública/Pan American Journal of Public Health*, 3, 9–14.

Oestergaard, M.Z., Inoue, M., Yoshida, S., Mahanani, W.R., Gore, F.M., Cousens, S., Lawn, J.E. & Mathers, C.D. 2011. Neonatal mortality levels for 193 countries in 2009 with trends since 1990: a systematic analysis of progress, projections, and priorities. *PLoS Medicine*, 8, e1001080.

Persson, L.A., Nga, N.T., Målqvist, M., Thi Phuong Hoa, D., Eriksson, L., Wallin, L., et al. 2013. Effect of facilitation of local maternal-and-newborn stakeholder groups on neonatal mortality: cluster-randomized controlled trial. *PLoS Medicine*, 10, e1001445.

Prost, A., Colbourn, T., Seward, N., Azad, K., Coomarasamy, A., Copas, A., et al. 2013. Women's groups practising participatory learning and action to improve maternal and newborn health in low-resource settings: a systematic review and meta-analysis. *Lancet*, 381, 1736–46.

Rajaratnam, J.K., Marcus, J.R., Flaxman, A.D., Wang, H., Levin-Rector, A., Dwyer, L., et al. 2010. Neonatal, postneonatal, childhood, and under-5 mortality for 187 countries, 1970–2010: a systematic analysis of progress towards Millennium Development Goal 4. *Lancet*, 375, 1988–2008.

Rosato, M., Laverack, G., Grabman, L.H., Tripathy, P., Nair, N., Mwansambo, C., et al. 2008. Community participation: lessons for maternal, newborn, and child health. *Lancet*, 372, 962–71.

Rycroft-Malone, J. 2004. The PARIHS framework – a framework for guiding the implementation of evidence-based practice. *Journal of Nursing Care Quality*, 19, 297–304.

Rycroft-Malone, J., Kitson, A., Harvey, G., McCormack, B., Seers, K., Titchen, A. & Estabrooks, C. 2002. Ingredients for change: revisiting a conceptual framework. *Quality and Safety in Health Care*, 11, 174–80.

Rycroft-Malone, J., Seers, K., Crichton, N., Chandler, J., Hawkes, C., Allen, C., Bullock, I. & Strunin, L. 2012. A pragmatic cluster randomised trial evaluating three implementation interventions. *Implementation Science*, 7, 80.

Save the Children 2013. *Surviving the First Day – State of the World's Mothers 2013.* London: Save the Children.

Scotland, G.S. & Bullough, C. H. 2004. What do doctors think their caseload should be to maintain their skills for delivery care? *International Journal of Gynecology and Obstetrics*, 87, 301–307.

Segall, M., Tipping, G., Lucas, H., Dung, T.V., Tam, N.T., Vinh, D.X. & Huong, D.L. 2002. Economic transition should come with a health warning: the case of Vietnam. *Journal of Epidemiology & Community Health*, 56, 497–505.

Stetler, C.B., Legro, M.W., Rycroft-Malone, J., Bowman, C., Curran, G., Guihan, M., et al. 2006. Role of 'external facilitation' in implementation of research findings: a qualitative evaluation of facilitation experiences in the Veterans Health Administration. *Implementation Science*, 1, 23.

Thompson, D.S., Estabrooks, C.A., Scott-Findlay, S., Moore, K. & Wallin, L. 2007. Interventions aimed at increasing research use in nursing: a systematic review. *Implementation Science*, 2, 15.

Thompson, G.N., Estabrooks, C.A. & Degner, L.F. 2006. Clarifying the concepts in knowledge transfer: a literature review. *Journal of Advanced Nursing*, 53, 691–701.

Tripathy, P., Nair, N., Barnett, S., Mahapatra, R., Borghi, J., Rath, S., et al. 2010. Effect of a participatory intervention with women's groups on birth outcomes and maternal depression in Jharkhand and Orissa, India: a cluster-randomised controlled trial. *Lancet*, 375, 1182–92.

UNICEF 2012. *The State of the World's Children.* New York: UNICEF.

United Nations 2006. *The Millennium Development Goals Report 2008.* New York: United Nations.

United Nations General Assembly 2000. *Resolution 2 session 55 United Nations Millennium Declaration.* New York: United Nations.

Wallin, L. 2009. Knowledge translation and implementation research in nursing. *International Journal of Nursing Studies*, 46, 576–87.

Wallin, L., Profetto-McGrath, J. & Levers, M.J. 2005a. Implementing nursing practice guidelines: a complex undertaking. *Journal of Wound Ostomy & Continence Nursing*, 32, 294–300; discussion 300–301.

Wallin, L., Rudberg, A. & Gunningberg, L. 2005b. Staff experiences in implementing guidelines for kangaroo mother care – a qualitative study. *International Journal of Nursing Studies*, 42, 61–73.

Wallin, L., Malqvist, M., Nga, N.T., Eriksson, L., Persson, L.A., Hoa, D.P., et al. 2011. Implementing knowledge into practice for improved neonatal survival; a cluster-randomised, community-based trial in Quang Ninh province, Vietnam. *BMC Health Services Research*, 11, 239.

Witter, S. 1996. 'Doi moi' and health: the effect of economic reforms on the health system in Vietnam. *International Journal of Health Planning and Management*, 11, 159–72.

Witter, S., Thi Thu Ha, B., Shengalia, B. & Vujicic, M. 2011. Understanding the 'four directions of travel': qualitative research into the factors affecting recruitment and retention of doctors in rural Vietnam. *Human Resources for Health*, 9, 20.

World Bank 2012. *Countries and Economies* [Online]. Available: http://data.worldbank.org/country [accessed 18 January 2012].

World Health Organization 2001. *Legal Status of Traditional Medicine and Complementary/Alternative Medicine: A Worldwide Review.* Geneva, Switzerland: World Health Organization.

World Health Organization 2002. *WHO Traditional Medicine Strategy 2002–2005.* Geneva: World Health Organization.

World Health Organization 2003. *Health and Ethnic Minorities in Viet Nam. Technical series No. 1.* Hanoi: World Health Organization.

World Health Organization 2011. *World Health Statistics.* Geneva: World Health Organization.

11

CASE STUDY OF THE PROWL PROJECT – A WHOLE-SYSTEM IMPLEMENTATION PROJECT INVOLVING NURSING AND DIETETIC LEAD FACILITATORS

Rick Wiechula, Alison Shanks, Tim Schultz, Nancy Whitaker and Alison Kitson

Introduction and background to the facilitation project

This case study presents a project conducted within a large tertiary hospital in Australia which aimed to improve the care and outcomes for older adults at risk of malnutrition. As with many such projects there was a dual purpose of improving practice but also adding to the science of knowledge translation. We used a staggered approach known as the stepped wedge design which allowed the project to be rolled out to a large number of wards as a staged process. This assisted with the logistical and practical issues that are encountered with such a large study (Hussey and Hughes, 2007). Four teams each with the responsibility of managing six to seven wards were established. We provide an overview of the project including the impetus to conduct the study and a detailed description of the study design and facilitation strategies. We include a description of the interventions that were used and evaluation of both processes and outcomes. The chapter concludes with a discussion of the lessons learnt, particularly with regard to the stepped wedge design and the advantages of working with experienced local facilitators.

Consequences of malnutrition

Older adults are at high risk of losing weight during a hospital admission (McWhirter and Pennington, 1994). This results in a range of significant adverse clinical outcomes, including pressure ulcers, functional decline, infections, increased re-admissions and mortality rates (Larsson, 1993; Klein et al., 1997; Covinsky et al., 1999; Kagansky et al., 2005; Mudge et al., 2011). Feeding patients in hospitals has become a widely recognised international problem with key deficits identified relating to issues of clinical ownership, increased frailty of patients, best use of resources and coordination of the hospital's dual roles of accommodating and treating patients (McWhirter and Pennington, 1994; Middleton et al., 2001; Watterson et al., 2009; Thibault et al., 2011).

The project 'Prevention and Reduction of Weight Loss (PRoWL) in the Acute Care Setting' notably builds on previous knowledge translation activities within the same hospital

(Kitson et al., 2013). Improving nutritional care and preventing weight loss of patients were identified by administrators and clinicians at the study hospital as key elements to improving the safety and quality of patient care. The Dietetic Department had been trialling malnutrition screening and assessment in a series of projects. Prior to the PRoWL collaboration, each of these professional groups and food services wished that the other two groups would do more for patient nutrition and felt that they could not achieve change; the patients fell through the gaps between the services. However, recent knowledge translation projects around nutrition screening and documentation had resulted in measurable improvement in two hospital wards. This activity also highlighted considerable interest in dealing with nutritional status in vulnerable patients throughout the organisation (Wiechula et al., 2009; Kitson et al., 2011). The hospital's internal auditing indicated that up to half of inpatients were at risk of nutritional decline.

Screening for malnutrition – the evidence base

We conducted a literature review to identify the potential elements of an intervention to prevent nutritional decline of patients in hospitals. Aside from having an evidence base to support the intervention, other necessary characteristics of the intervention were that: it was feasible to implement across the hospital, it involved multiple disciplines (food services, dietetics and nursing), it was inexpensive, and that known local barriers to best practice in nutritional decline were addressed.

The literature search identified three broad groups of interventions used in hospitals to prevent nutritional decline: using a structured tool to screen for malnutrition, provision of additional nutritional supplements, and assistance with feeding (Kitson et al., 2013). The specific evidence base behind each element of the intervention is described in more detail elsewhere (Kitson et al., 2013).

The literature review identified a number of intervention studies that had sought to prevent nutritional decline of 'at-risk' patients, with mixed results. By and large these studies focused only on a single intervention, which targeted a single healthcare profession and a particular sub-set of patients. The novelty of the PRoWL project was that it combined a number of elements into a multi-faceted, multi-disciplinary intervention that was delivered across virtually the entire hospital (Kitson et al., 2013).

Overview of the facilitation approach adopted

In considering the facilitation approach used in the project this section will describe the two aspects of facilitation. First, we will describe who the facilitators were and then the process of facilitation that was used (Figure 11.1). Although we had previously conducted projects within this organisation and used many similar strategies, there were some significant differences with this project in terms of who was providing the facilitation and how it was managed.

External facilitators

The project used both external and internal facilitators. There existed a very long-term relationship between the acute care teaching hospital where the project took place and the university that provided the external facilitation (ALK and RW). Indeed the two organisations

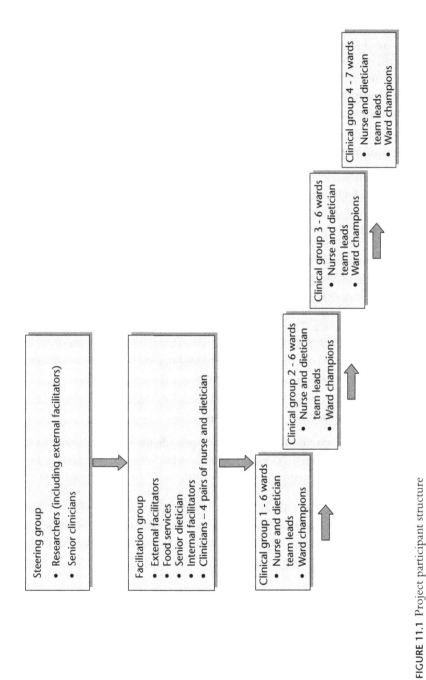

FIGURE 11.1 Project participant structure

are co-located on the same site. The two external facilitators were familiar with the hospital and the staff who were recruited as internal facilitators. Both had been involved in previous implementation projects at the site and indeed one of the external facilitators had been a senior clinician within the hospital a number of years previously. In addition to the external facilitators who worked directly with the internal facilitation team, the project was supported by a team of researchers and senior clinicians who formed a project steering group. This group contained researchers with experience in nutritional science and knowledge translation. They assisted the internal facilitation team with analysis and reporting of audit data and also collected additional data relating to weight loss of the patients involved. The researchers also collected data in relation to the facilitation aspects of the project. The intent was not only to conduct an implementation project but also to add to the body of evidence in relation to implementation.

Internal facilitators

The internal facilitators for this project were volunteers. The recruitment targeted senior clinicians from both dietetics and nursing. The project involved 25 wards divided into four groups (three groups of 6 and one of 7). Each of the four teams was led by two internal facilitators. One was a senior nurse in charge of one of the wards within their group and the other a dietician. The facilitation team was rounded out with the Head of Dietetics (AS) and the Head of Food Services and the two external facilitators. Although it was not a specific inclusion criterion for the internal facilitators, a number of these clinicians, both dieticians and nurses, had been involved in knowledge translation projects previously, either with the external facilitators or as part of the Joanna Briggs Institute Clinical Leaders Program (http://joannabriggs.org/jbi-education.html). The local facilitators also recruited champions in each of the wards they had been allocated. They did this by working through the senior nurse clinicians on the wards. The ward champions did not have to be senior clinicians but it was important that they had the support of the wards' most senior nurse.

Facilitation processes and timelines

The role of the external facilitators was to provide the necessary support to the internal facilitators and act as liaison between the facilitation team and the steering group. The external facilitators were not expected to lead the project but to provide whatever support was needed by the internal facilitators throughout the project. This varied from advice about accessing evidence to strategies for working with the ward champions. It also included assistance with audit tool design and analysis of results. The level and nature of the facilitation was tailored to the internal facilitators' needs. An important first step was to establish what experience the internal facilitators had with implementation projects. In our previous projects considerable time was spent training the internal facilitators in various aspects of implementation. Notably with this group of internal facilitators, formal training was minimal because of their previous experience; therefore, planning of the project was able to commence more quickly than with previous projects. Monthly meetings were held with the facilitation team. At the first meeting it was important to negotiate the ground rules. In particular the discussions at the monthly meetings were to be confidential. The internal facilitators worked with the steering group to identify a range of potential interventions that could be implemented during the project. In considering which of the interventions would be used, the facilitation group considered the evidence to support the interventions and the contextual issues that would indicate their appropriateness and feasibility. The interventions that were adopted are detailed below. Although a number of the local facilitators were experienced with knowledge translation work there was still a reasonably long preparatory phase prior to implementation commencing.

Preliminary meetings with what would become the steering group began in August of 2010. The steering group met monthly until well into the implementation phase. The facilitation group began monthly meetings in February of 2011. By the February meeting the overall design and structure of the project had been finalised and the facilitation group then met to do detailed planning regarding implementation. Implementation began in April of 2011 and the plan was for successive teams to commence at two-monthly intervals. All groups had conducted the implementation by December of 2012 and the final round of data collection for the project occurred in mid-2013.

Implementing the evidence: project design

Within the overall facilitation framework there were three main interventions targeted to improve the nutritional status of older adults. As previously discussed it is important to identify those patients at risk of malnutrition. Although there are many screening tools available it was decided by the group that the Malnutrition Universal Screening Tool (MUST) (Elia, 2003) would be implemented. The dietetics staff were familiar with MUST, which had been used previously in the hospital, however in only a small number of units. The tool was considered appropriate because it can be completed fairly rapidly and does not require patients to be weighed if reliable data can be provided by the patient or relative (Stratton et al., 2004, 2006; Lamb et al., 2009). Once patients were identified as being at risk of malnutrition they were to have oral nutritional supplements provided to them (NICE, 2006; Stratton and Elia, 2007; Vanderkroft et al., 2007). These were in the form of pre-packaged milk- or juice-based drinks. From previous internal auditing at the hospital it was known that many patients who required assistance with feeding were not getting that assistance in a timely fashion, with meal trays often being removed from the patient without the meal being eaten. The third intervention therefore was the introduction of red trays. These highly visual trays would be allocated to patients who required assistance with feeding. This was a visual cue for both the nursing staff who were required to provide the assistance but also the food services staff who manage the delivery and return of meal trays (Bradley and Rees, 2003; Bradley, 2006; Davis, 2007). These three key interventions were largely new initiatives but a number of existing interventions were also modified and given renewed focus. For example, there was an existing nutritional observation chart that was reviewed and updated. Signage placed above the bedheads to indicate dietary requirements was also modified to include an indicator that a red tray would be used.

An important element of the implementation process was the education of all staff about the interventions being implemented. In order to manage this education effectively across 25 wards a 'train the trainer' system was adopted. The facilitation group planned and developed the education package with the assistance of the external facilitators. Folders with all the education materials were supplied to each ward. The local facilitators then trained the ward champions who in turn trained the ward staff. The advantage of the staged approach was that the burden of removing clinical staff for training was spread over many months, with each group of wards completing the bulk of the training before the next group commenced. Using this train the trainer approach eight trainers became nearly 50 trainers. In addition, the dieticians undertook an extensive training programme for the food services staff who would be dealing with the red trays.

Prior to the implementation phase of the project clinical audits were carried out on the wards. The audits were repeated after the implementation phase and then a final audit at the end of the project was conducted in all wards.

Methods used to identify and work with stakeholders

The scope of the project and the focus of the implementation strategies meant that the stakeholders for the project were quite diverse. Although some specialist units within the hospital were not involved in the project, the majority of inpatient wards were. As a result, support for the project was required from the Director of Nursing and the Nursing Directors of each division within the hospital. The nurses in charge of the individual wards were also considered key as they were required to identify the champions for their wards and provide them with ongoing support. The nature of the project meant that large numbers of clinicians needed to be aware of what was going on. This included the majority of the nursing establishment, dieticians and food services staff.

A communication strategy was planned from the beginning of the project. Hospital-wide forums were used to introduce the project and then follow-up sessions provided to update on progress as the project continued. The Director of Nursing received regular briefings and the project was on the agenda of the nursing executives' meetings. Regular updates in newsletters which reached across the area health service where the hospital was situated were provided. This not only kept the hospital staff informed but generated considerable interest in the project from other hospitals in the city facing similar issues.

Methods used to assess and respond to contextual issues

Using the principles embodied in the PARIHS framework (Kitson et al., 1998), several processes were used in our facilitation approach to deal with the myriad contextual issues that arise within a large organisation. In addition, although it was not intended as a facilitation strategy, the stepped wedge design also had some positive impacts on the facilitation of the project. This is essentially an experimental design that allows for a number of groups to initially be enrolled as controls and in a staged fashion each control group in turn then crosses over to receive the intervention (Hussey and Hughes, 2007). The decision to use this design was based on the need to ensure robustness in relation to the measurement of outcomes. Each group or step acts as its own control. This design is well suited to interventions implemented in large complex organisations where a staged roll-out is more practical and manageable (Kitson et al., 2013). It is used where there is confidence that the intervention will be beneficial and therefore no group is left without receiving the intervention at some point in the study (Brown and Lilford, 2006; Hussey and Hughes, 2007; Brown et al., 2008).

We had four teams each led by a dietician and a nurse. The team leads (local facilitators) were responsible for managing the implementation in a number of wards. The nurse lead was the senior registered nurse in one of the wards within their group. Group 1 began implementation in

April of 2011. Subsequent groups commenced implementation at approximately two-monthly intervals (Table 11.1). It was apparent from the beginning of the study that contextual issues were going to be encountered at a ward, division and organisation level. The stepped wedge design meant that as the project was rolled out contextual issues could be identified in the first group and the facilitation strategy modified accordingly (Kitson et al., 2013). The three elements of the complex intervention – MUST, nourishing fluids and the red trays – remained constant but logistical and practical issues in providing these elements were dealt with as they arose. The facilitation group met monthly throughout the project. This allowed for the groups that had commenced implementation to discuss issues directly with those about to commence. This underlines the importance that we had placed on peer support within this group. The issues that did arise were many and varied. For example, when the first group commenced they were able to discuss with the others in the facilitation group how best to deal with the ward champions. The ward champions were selected by the individual ward's senior clinical nurse. The nurse team leaders were therefore familiar with and had much more direct contact with the champions on their own wards; however, with the other wards in their group they were, to a degree, outsiders. They had to spend a great deal more time getting to know the ward champions and ensuring they felt supported than they had initially expected. It also became apparent that the relationship with the champions was impacted greatly by the local nurse leaders in the wards. In some wards the champions may have been very enthusiastic while the nurse leader was somewhat resistant.

Other issues arose that were clearly organisation-wide. Having nourishing fluids available was identified as a very complex issue. Appropriate fridges needed to be available on the wards. Stock management required significant negotiation with the supply department. Stock rotation needed to be managed. Who would be responsible to pay for the drinks became an issue in an organisation with tight budgets. Negotiation between food services, the materials supply department and the clinicians managed to overcome these issues in the spirit of collaboration and joint responsibility for an issue that was recognised as a priority. The stepped wedge design also guided the timing of our data collection. We collected baseline data using a structured clinical audit tool to measure compliance with the project interventions. The team leads worked with the local champions to undertake the audits. Baseline audits were conducted just prior to implementation. Follow-up audits were conducted two months after the implementation and again for all groups at the end of the project.

In addition to the baseline audit we also used the Alberta Context Tool (ACT), which measures aspects of organisational context that can influence the implementation of evidence

TABLE 11.1 Stepped wedge design timeline

Stage Group/ Step	1	2	3	4	5	6
1. Wards 1–6	0; ACT	X	P			P
2. Wards 7–12		0; ACT	X	P		P
3. Wards 13–18			0; ACT	X	P	P
4. Wards 19–25				0; ACT	X	P

Abbreviation: 0, baseline data collection; ACT, Alberta Context Tool; X, intervention and data collection; P, post-intervention data collection.

in to practice (Estabrooks et al., 2009). Our aim was to use ACT to enable local facilitators to consider any strengths or hindrances that might impact on the project implementation. The tool measures staff views regarding leadership, culture, feedback processes, connections among people, staff, space and time (Estabrooks et al., 2009; Schultz and Kitson, 2010). The ACT was designed to measure these parameters at an organisational level but we also analysed the results at a unit level. Our intent was that the team leads would feedback the results to the nurses in charge of the individual wards. However, the local facilitators were uncomfortable with undertaking such direct feedback and only considered the results more broadly.

Evaluating the impact of facilitation

The impact of the project was judged in a number of ways. In the first instance we wanted to establish the effectiveness of the intervention in preventing nutritional decline of patients. The results indicated some reduction in nutritional decline in the second week of the hospital stay, although the sample size was lower than expected, limiting the statistical power to detect a difference at this time period (Schultz et al., 2014). Second, we wanted to assess the degree of uptake of all the project interventions through analysing the local audit data. Acknowledging the complexity of the intervention, we also wanted to understand the impact on those directly involved in the project.

In conducting the audits, champions in each ward selected a convenience sample of 10 patients for each audit round. As older adults had previously been identified as a vulnerable group, patients over 65 were specifically targeted. In keeping with the trajectory of care the first audit questions were around screening. Use of MUST had an overall baseline of compliance of 17%. Although for most wards this was a completely new intervention, there were a small number of wards that had previously used the tool. Following implementation, the overall compliance rate was 51% and at the end of the project this moved to 59% compliance. Figure 11.2 provides results for each of the four groups and the overall result for all wards combined.

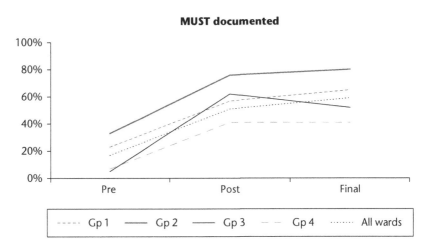

FIGURE 11.2 Compliance rates with MUST documentation

The hospital did already have the capacity to provide a range of nourishing fluids. However, prior to the project commencing, the mechanism to obtain supplies was considered cumbersome and in most wards there was no ongoing stock available. Special orders needed to be made through the stores which took considerable time. The provision of nutritional supplements for those identified at risk of nutritional decline had an overall baseline of 10% compliance. This moved to 55% after implementation and at project end had dipped slightly to 44% (Figure 11.3).

The intervention that created the most attention, largely because of its visual and novel nature, was the use of red trays for those requiring full assistance with feeding. The use of the red trays began at a baseline of 4% and moved to 40% post implementation, rising further to 52% compliance at project end. Although there was overall improvement in this measure, the results did vary across wards and groups, as seen in Figure 11.4. Group 3 had a relatively high

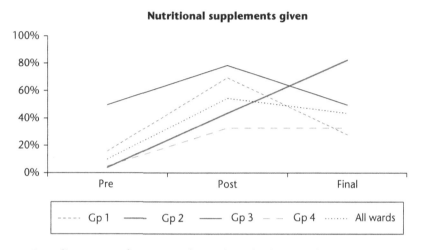

FIGURE 11.3 Compliance rates of provision of nourishing fluids to at-risk patients

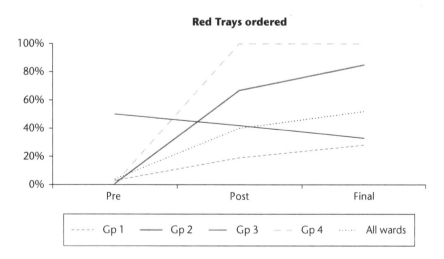

FIGURE 11.4 Compliance rates of provision of red trays

baseline measure of compliance and investigation determined some crossover had occurred by the time they commenced implementation. It is the nature of large acute care hospitals that there will be a good deal of staff movement between units both on a shift-by-shift basis and more permanently.

For all three measures there were clear improvements that were mostly sustained through to the end of the project. We did not formally set target compliance rates at the beginning of the project and only one group achieved 100% compliance on one measure, the red trays. Despite this, the local facilitators were pleased with the overall improvements.

In addition to the audits of practice, we collected data from and about the facilitators. This included information from the monthly meetings, the electronic communications within the facilitation group and then finally formal interviews with each of the local facilitators. As discussed previously, a number of the local facilitators had previous experience with similar projects. Those with prior experience highlighted the importance of building on the skills and knowledge they already possessed. Those with less experience commented on the value of the peer support and advice provided by the more experienced local facilitators. Some of the facilitators with less experience indicated they were somewhat unsure initially what was expected of them but as the monthly team meetings progressed the peer support assisted them to gain a firm sense of where they fitted within the project. The facilitators spoke of gaining confidence through the project. As external facilitators we were aware that these clinicians were being placed at some risk with regard to their reputation. The monthly meetings meant there was considerable scrutiny from their peers in relation to each team's progress. Considerable effort was put in place to ensure discussions at the monthly meetings were confidential and reinforced a no-blame culture. Mistakes were declared with the purpose of adapting the implementation strategy and moving the project forward to benefit all of the teams.

The communication strategy also called for reporting of the project's progress at various organisational forums. It was obvious at the forums that the internal facilitators were increasing in confidence as the project progressed, particularly when they were able to report improvements in practice. Although not a stated objective, the project was an opportunity for participants to get to know other staff in the hospital who they would not normally deal with. This occurred between the local facilitators and the ward champions, but even more apparent were the relationships with the other facilitators. There was a strong sense of camaraderie within the facilitation group and they particularly spoke of having a much better understanding of the other discipline's role and a growing appreciation of their part in ensuring the nutritional requirements of patients were met.

From the beginning of the project it was overtly stated that any initiatives that could improve the nutritional status of the patients should be long term and be sustained beyond the life of the project. In particular it was felt important that there needed to be better awareness of the roles and responsibilities of all those involved. Early discussions with the facilitation group indicated there had been an historical shift in how meals were provided to patients. In years past food was delivered to wards and the nursing staff distributed the meals to the patients. Some years prior to this project the responsibility of giving meal trays directly to the patients passed to the food services staff. This unintentionally created a disconnect between the simple act of placing a tray before the patient and the responsibility of ensuring patients had the nutrition they required. The facilitation group felt it was important that nurses within the organisation regained the sense that nutrition was a fundamental aspect of care which they were primarily responsible for. This was reflected in the education packages and the communication activities throughout the project. Local data from previous projects showing that 48% of patients were either malnourished or at medium to high risk of malnutrition provided salient messages. As the project progressed there was a growing sense of ownership of this issue from the local facilitators and the ward champions. They felt empowered to take the issue on and were encouraged that most nurses were happy to support the project.

As the project neared completion there was active planning to ensure the responsibility to monitor activity and indeed to keep things improving was handed over to the organisation. Further strategies have been used to embed the PRoWL interventions into practice. Auditing of rates of malnutrition screening, provision of nourishing fluids, monitoring of intake and referral of high-risk patients for dietetic review has been built into the routine audit schedule of the fundamentals of nursing care, with the results fed back to each ward. This has demonstrated that rates of screening have not only been maintained but are improving. In January 2014 audit results indicated that 98% of patients had nutrition and hydration assessed and documented on admission. In relation to MUST specifically, two years after the formal completion of the project the compliance rate of MUST completion on admission was 68%. The auditing programme examines rates of dietetic referral for patients at high risk and these continue to increase. All this indicates an increasing recognition of the essential nature of nutritional care within the organisation and as a result the nursing, dietetic and food services staff have continued to support other nutrition-related improvements such as decreasing unnecessary fasting and improving patient hydration.

Reflections and lessons learnt

The clinical focus for this project was singular. The aim was to improve nutrition of patients across the organisation. In previous projects where we have used multiple teams of local facilitators we have allowed teams to select different aspects of care for their improvement project. What resulted were projects of much smaller scope where each project presented the local and external facilitators with unique problems to solve. The ability to learn from the other teams involved and pool resources to solve common problems was diminished. The focus on a single aspect of care – nutritional support – made best use of the staggered approach of the project.

The stepped wedge design was initially adopted because it was considered an efficient but robust method to measure the effectiveness of introducing an intervention in a complex system. The added advantage of the design was the ability to deal with logistical and practical issues of a large project while still maintaining a structured approach to implementing the interventions. This allowed a degree of flexibility in terms of adjusting the facilitation strategy between groups. For example, when issues arose that required an organisation-wide solution others in the facilitation group could act to assist. A strong principle that we have used for our knowledge translation projects is the need to be flexible and adapt facilitation in order to manage unforeseen issues that arise while still keeping within a structure that maintains the integrity of the evaluation. However, the flexibility of the project, in terms of the ability to modify the intervention between groups, raises issues about the fidelity of the intervention within the context of an experimental design.

A further reflection relates to the fact that the length of the preparatory phase should not be underestimated. Getting a good understanding of the potential contextual issues is extremely important. Getting to know the local facilitators and what their needs are is equally important. Having a clear sense that senior management of the organisation will champion the project is mandatory. Once the project commenced it was critical that the facilitation had a structure to work within. Although flexibility is seen to be valuable this does not mean that anything goes. From the beginning of the project timelines and goals were set. Any changes to the plan had to be well justified. There was some movement in the timelines, which, to a degree, must be expected when working with a large organisation that is dynamic in nature. The one downside to the structure of the stepped wedge design was the frustration felt by the last group to commence implementation. The project had a very high profile due to the scope of the project and the deliberate communication strategies used. The staff in the wards from the last group placed a great deal of pressure on the local facilitators to get going ahead of the scheduled start.

As discussed, the external facilitators had conducted previous knowledge translation projects at this hospital. This had a number of important advantages. The external facilitators were known to both the senior management of the organisation and importantly to the local facilitators they were going to be working directly with. It is important that those involved in this type of project are aware of everyone's roles and responsibilities and that there is a level of trust that each member of the team is able to deliver. The external facilitators' knowledge of the organisation assisted in defining the scope of the project and understanding some of the potential contextual issues that may be problematic. Having experienced local facilitators was also a considerable advantage. We felt this assisted with the preparatory phase but also with the peer support they provided to the inexperienced facilitators throughout the project. This situation did not develop by chance. The willingness to develop a long-term partnership through these projects is felt by both the external facilitators from the university and the senior nurses of the hospital. The intent is to build capacity within the hospital to undertake such projects and from the academics' perspective to further the science of knowledge translation. Over time, the outsiders from the university have become virtual insiders within the hospital.

When the project was set up it was agreed that there would be two leaders for each team and they would be from nursing and dietetics. This decision was both symbolic and practical. It was symbolic as the message to the hospital staff was one of shared responsibility for nutrition. In a practical sense it meant that there was sufficient spread of knowledge and skill in each team and that there would be back-up if one team lead was not available. In line with this, we also encouraged the team leads to recruit at least two champions on each ward to provide mutual support and back-up. In some cases they were only able to recruit one staff member and in others even two were not sufficient to get through the project. We received feedback from some of the team leads that the process of co-facilitation was not sufficiently explained at the start of the project. They felt that others were doing more and that the load was inequitable. The lesson for the external facilitators is to be vigilant about how the teams are functioning and although a number were experienced in conducting these projects, assumptions need to be explored and verified.

Sustainability is not always considered with knowledge translation projects, but the investment of those involved dictates it should be a priority and planned as part of the project. The relationships between the different disciplines have continued to grow beyond the project and further initiatives have been put in place. At the time of writing another project focusing on hydration has commenced with external facilitators from the university and local facilitators, some of whom were involved in the PRoWL project. The ward champions have also continued to support nutritional care. There has necessarily needed to be further recruitment of champions but the role is now embedded in all wards. Ongoing monitoring and evaluation has been taken on through the existing hospital audit programme.

What this case study adds to our overall understanding of facilitation

Balance of flexibility and structure

Our experience over a number of projects conducted either in large organisations or with multiple organisations during the same project is that despite allowing for an extended preparatory phase there will always be issues arising during the project that are unforeseen and may impact significantly on the success of the project. There is, therefore, usually a need to adapt the facilitation strategy. This is balanced against the need to have detailed planning that provides structure and guidance to the project. This is particularly important in knowledge translation projects where outcomes are often difficult to attribute to the interventions and the implementation strategies used. This has resonance with the debate about pragmatic and explanatory trial designs. Pragmatic trials are conducted in real-life contexts where interventions are delivered with a degree of flexibility, recognising that is how care is often delivered (Patsopoulos, 2011).

Capacity building

This project was not conducted in isolation and is one of a series of knowledge translation projects conducted in partnership between the university and the hospital. This project illustrates the advantages of an ongoing relationship that has resulted in increased understanding and trust between the organisations and, most importantly, availability of a large number of experienced local facilitators. Care needs to be taken to ensure the local facilitators are supported in relation to their individual needs but it is clearly an advantage to begin a project where local facilitators have an understanding about what their own role is and that of the external facilitators. In keeping with the notion of capacity building there was a mix of experienced and less experienced facilitators; the latter learning from and being supported by the former. The strategy we use is to have the facilitation group meet regularly and emphasise from the beginning the notions of collegiality and mutual support.

The notion of capacity building is equally important for the external facilitators. Our School now has a number of academics, bringing a range of skills, knowledge and experience in knowledge translation. We always conduct projects within teams, encouraging less experienced staff to work with our more experienced facilitators. We are committed to formally investigating and evaluating each project not only to increase our own capacity but to add to the body of evidence for knowledge translation.

Awareness of reputational risk

The local facilitators for this project were all reasonably senior clinicians. They were used to working in multi-disciplinary teams, managing staff and solving clinical problems. They all had a detailed understanding of the system they worked in and were familiar with being judged on their performance. All this would suggest they would be comfortable in the role of a facilitator for a knowledge translation project. Even for the local facilitators with prior experience this was a significant assumption. In conducting a hospital-wide initiative there is a level of scrutiny that goes beyond their day-to-day practice. As part of our facilitation we build into each project a communications strategy. Success for these types of projects relies on convincing many people in the organisation of the value of the project. This raises the level of scrutiny for our clinical partners often to a very uncomfortable level. They are judged by their peers on the success of the project and by the management that is providing the resource to conduct the project. It is imperative then for external facilitators to provide a supportive environment and not underestimate the level of exposure the local facilitators may experience.

Sustainability

All projects run the risk of a loss of momentum when they come to an end. External facilitation for the work is usually withdrawn and gains in improved care can fade unless long-term strategies are put in place. In this project many of the strategies used required system-wide change. These changes are the most difficult to implement because it often requires assistance or agreement from those not directly involved or invested in the project. In this project system changes that needed to be made were identified as early as possible and the necessary stakeholders engaged. This was assisted by the communications strategy. An example is the MUST which had been used previously in a few small projects. When we commenced our project we needed to have the MUST available electronically and were able to have it placed on the hospital intranet. The long-term solution, however, was to have the MUST assessment included in the admission documentation. This occurred at a time when the entire health system was moving from a paper-based to an electronic patient record system. The success of the project helped to ensure the MUST was included in the new system. The lesson was to commence sustainability planning within and not at the end of the project.

This project was in many ways an exercise in compromise. Like other projects we have undertaken there are a series of balancing acts that need to be considered and agreed to. There is a balance between the needs and goals of the clinicians and the researchers. Clinicians will largely be concerned with getting on with the job of improving care. The researchers are concerned with adding to the science of knowledge translation. The study design needs to be robust to demonstrate the impact of the intervention while being flexible enough to accommodate the shifting realities of real-world practice. The success of this project was in understanding the shared goal of improving nutrition in this vulnerable group. The clinicians from different disciplines, the researchers, the service staff and the hospital management all understood this goal and the shared sense of responsibility. This allowed the necessary balances in the project to be achieved.

References

Bradley, L. 2006. Red trays for people at nutritional risk have boosted patient satisfaction. *Nursing Standard*, 21, 30–1.

Bradley, L. & Rees, C. 2003. Reducing nutritional risk in hospital: the red tray. *Nursing Standard*, 17, 33–7.

Brown, C.A. & Lilford, R.J. 2006. The stepped wedge trial design: a systematic review. *BMC Medical Research Methodology*, 6.

Brown, C., Hofer, T., Johal, A., Thomson, R., Nicholl, J., Franklin, B.D. & Lilford, R.J. 2008. An epistemology of patient safety research: A framework for study design and interpretation. Part 2. Study design. *Quality and Safety in Health Care*, 17, 163–9.

Covinsky, K.E., Martin, G.E., Beyth, R.J., Justice, A.C., Sehgal, A.R. & Landefeld, C.S. 1999. The relationship between clinical assessments of nutritional status and adverse outcomes in older hospitalized medical patients. *Journal of the American Geriatrics Society*, 47, 532–8.

Davis, C. 2007. Mealtime solutions. *Nursing Standard*, 21, 21–3.

Elia, M. 2003. *The 'MUST', Report. Nutritional Screening for Adults: A Multidisciplinary Responsibility. Development and use of the 'Malnutrition Universal Screening Tool', (MUST) for adults.* British Association for Parenteral and Enteral Nutrition (BAPEN).

Estabrooks, C.A., Squires, J.E., Cummings, G.G., Birdsell, J.M. & Norton, P.G. 2009. Development and assessment of the Alberta Context Tool. *BMC Health Services Research*, 9.

Hussey, M.A. & Hughes, J.P. 2007. Design and analysis of stepped wedge cluster randomized trials. *Contemporary Clinical Trials*, 28, 182–91.

Kagansky, N., Berner, Y., Koren-Morag, N., Perelman, L., Knobler, H. & Levy, S. 2005. Poor nutritional habits are predictors of poor outcome in very old hospitalized patients. *American Journal of Clinical Nutrition*, 82, 784–91; quiz 913–14.

Kitson, A., Harvey, G. & McCormack, B. 1998. Enabling the implementation of evidence based practice: a conceptual framework. *Quality in Health Care*, 7, 149–58.

Kitson, A., Silverston, H., Wiechula, R., Zeitz, K., Marcoionni, D. & Page, T. 2011. Clinical nursing leaders', team members' and service managers' experiences of implementing evidence at a local level. *Journal of Nursing Management*, 19, 542–55.

Kitson, A.L., Schultz, T.J., Long, L., Shanks, A., Wiechula, R., Chapman, I. & Soenen, S. 2013. The prevention and reduction of weight loss in an acute tertiary care setting: protocol for a pragmatic stepped wedge randomised cluster trial (the PRoWL project). *BMC Health Services Research*, 13, 299.

Klein, S., Kinney, J., Jeejeebhoy, K., Alpers, D., Hellerstein, M., Murray, M. & Twomey, P. 1997. Nutrition support in clinical practice: review of published data and recommendations for future research directions. National Institutes of Health, American Society for Parenteral and Enteral Nutrition, and American Society for Clinical Nutrition. *JPEN Journal of Parenteral and Enteral Nutrition*, 21, 133–56.

Lamb, C.A., Parr, J., Lamb, E.I. & Warren, M.D. 2009. Adult malnutrition screening, prevalence and management in a United Kingdom hospital: cross-sectional study. *British Journal of Nutrition*, 102, 571–5.

Larsson, J. 1993. Clinical problem of hospital malnutrition. *Nutrition*, 9, 274.

McWhirter, J.P. & Pennington, C.R. 1994. Incidence and recognition of malnutrition in hospital. *British Medical Journal*, 308, 945–8.

Middleton, M.H., Nazarenko, G., Nivison-Smith, I. & Smerdely, P. 2001. Prevalence of malnutrition and 12-month incidence of mortality in two Sydney teaching hospitals. *Internal Medicine Journal*, 31, 455–61.

Mudge, A.M., Kasper, K., Clair, A., Redfern, H., Bell, J.J., Barras, M.A., Dip, G. & Pachana, N.A. 2011. Recurrent readmissions in medical patients: a prospective study. *Journal of Hospital Medicine*, 6, 61–7.

NICE (National Institute for Health and Clinical Excellence) 2006. *Nutrition Support for Adults: Oral Nutrition Support, Enteral Tube Feeding and Parenteral Nutrition*. London: NICE.

Patsopoulos, N.A. 2011. A pragmatic view on pragmatic trials. *Dialogues in Clinical Neuroscience*, 13, 217–24.

Schultz, T., Kitson, A., Soenen, S., Long, L., Shanks, A., Wiechula, R., Chapman, I. & Lange, K. 2014. Does a multidisciplinary nutritional intervention prevent nutritional decline in hospital patients? A stepped wedge randomised cluster trial. *e-SPEN Journal*, 9, e84–e90.

Schultz, T.J. & Kitson, A.L. 2010. Measuring the context of care in an Australian acute care hospital: a nurse survey. *Implementation Science*, 5.

Stratton, R.J. & Elia, M. 2007. A review of reviews: A new look at the evidence for oral nutritional supplements in clinical practice. *Clinical Nutrition*, Suppl 2, 5–23.

Stratton, R.J., Hackston, A., Longmore, D., Dixon, R., Price, S., Stroud, M., King, C. & Elia, M. 2004. Malnutrition in hospital outpatients and inpatients: prevalence, concurrent validity and ease of use of the 'malnutrition universal screening tool' ('MUST') for adults. *British Journal of Nutrition*, 92, 799–808.

Stratton, R.J., King, C.L., Stroud, M.A., Jackson, A.A. & Elia, M. 2006. 'Malnutrition Universal Screening Tool' predicts mortality and length of hospital stay in acutely ill elderly. *British Journal of Nutrition*, 95, 325–30.

Thibault, R., Chikhi, M., Clerc, A., Darmon, P., Chopard, P., Genton, L., Kossovsky, M.P. & Pichard, C. 2011. Assessment of food intake in hospitalised patients: a 10-year comparative study of a prospective hospital survey. *Clinical Nutrition*, 30, 289–96.

Vanderkroft, D., Collins, C.E., Fitzgerald, M., Lewis, S., Neve, M. & Capra, S. 2007. Minimising undernutrition in the older inpatient. *International Journal of Evidence-Based Healthcare*, 5, 110–81.

Watterson, C., Fraser, A., Banks, M., Isenring, E., Miller, M., Silvester, C., et al. 2009. Evidence based practice guidelines for the nutritional management of malnutrition in adult patients across the continuum of care. *Nutrition and Dietetics*, 66, S1–S34.

Wiechula, R., Kitson, A., Marcoionni, D., Page, T., Zeitz, K. & Silverston, H. 2009. Improving the fundamentals of care for older people in the acute hospital setting: facilitating practice improvement using a Knowledge Translation Toolkit. *International Journal of Evidence Based Healthcare*, 7, 283–95.

12

CASE STUDY OF THE SIGNATURE PROJECT – AN AUSTRALIAN–US KNOWLEDGE TRANSLATION PROJECT

Alison Kitson, Rick Wiechula, Tiff Conroy, Nancy Whitaker, Cheryl Holly and Susan Salmond

Introduction and background to the facilitation project

In 2010 a project was set up between two collaborating centres of the Joanna Briggs Institute (JBI). These were the Centre for Evidence Based Practice, South Australia (CEPSA) based in the University of Adelaide and the New Jersey Centre for Evidence Based Practice (NJCEBP), located within Rutgers University, formerly the University of Medicine and Dentistry New Jersey (UMDNJ). The project was known as 'The Signature Project' as all the participants 'signed up' to an 18-month knowledge translation (KT) project. The project involved a team of expert facilitators and researchers in South Australia, a team of academic facilitators and researchers in New Jersey and six clinical care sites located throughout New Jersey.

The primary objective of the project was to provide participants with first-hand experience of trying to implement a piece of new evidence into practice. In addition to this, the New Jersey Team wanted to strengthen and build partnerships between the university and the six organisations involved by assisting the participants to develop facilitation skills.

The primary aim of the Signature Project was to investigate how evidence is introduced into practice using a structured intervention, the Knowledge Translation (KT) Toolkit, which is based on expert facilitation and support. The KT Toolkit (Wiechula et al., 2009; Kitson et al., 2012) is derived from the Promoting Action on Research in Health Services (PARIHS) conceptual framework (Kitson et al., 1998, 2008). It was intended that this project would extend the body of evidence on what works in getting new evidence into practice and, in particular, influence the guidance and teaching materials for KT produced by JBI collaborating centres worldwide (over 90 centres in 60 countries) (Pearson et al., 2005). At the time no systematic investigation of facilitation as outlined in the PARIHS framework had been undertaken in the North American health system, although the Veterans Administration had selected PARIHS as one of the KT frameworks upon which to build its system-wide KT strategy (Stetler et al., 2006). The New Jersey sites agreed to be involved in testing the transferability of the PARIHS and KT theory and methods while working to improve patient care through the introduction of new evidence.

It is now widely acknowledged that the movement of existing evidence into everyday clinical practice is a challenging and complex task. There has been significant interest in, and uptake of, methods to appraise, review and synthesise original research evidence in such a way as to create suitable products for clinical practice. However there is still a lag between the production of such evidence and its implementation in clinical settings. For an international collaboration such as JBI, there has been significant effort put into understanding how collaborating centres can more systematically investigate this implementation gap. JBI has an approach to building capacity for the implementation of new evidence in health systems called the JBI Clinical Fellows programme. This programme brings together individuals from health systems across the world to train them in the basic skills of practice change: evidence appraisal, the development of standards and criteria based on the evidence, undertaking baseline audits, introducing a series of improvements and reauditing. Following a weeklong intensive programme, the fellows return home to undertake an improvement project based on a problem they wish to investigate. After a six-month period the fellows return to JBI to provide feedback on their progress and to generate an improvement report. Many of these studies have been published and illustrate how individuals can begin to shape practice by introducing evidence in a structured way.

What the Signature Project wanted to do was apply a more explicit KT facilitative approach to this step in the knowledge-to-action process. Instead of having individual clinicians come out of their health systems and undertake a period of study, the Signature Project aimed to establish a partnership between two JBI collaborating centres where the expertise and facilitation skills could be shared in a structured way. The South Australian Collaborating Centre staff were proficient in expert facilitation and evaluation research and the New Jersey Collaborating Center was eager to extend its impact across the local health systems by developing expertise in facilitating evidence-based practice.

Overview of the facilitation approach used

The facilitation approach used was based on expert external facilitators (the University of Adelaide team) supporting six novice external facilitators who were faculty members of UMDNJ and also members of the New Jersey JBI Collaborating Center. These six novice external facilitators were called academic coordinators (ACs) and their job was to partner with six local novice internal facilitators (IFs) from each of the six volunteer clinical sites or health systems (Figure 12.1).

Following a three-day KT training workshop, faculty ACs and health facility IFs were asked to identify the local interdisciplinary team with whom they would work over an 18-month period to introduce the new piece of evidence. Potential team members were to be told about the project and invited to participate. Those team members who wished to participate would then receive more detailed information about the expectations of the project.

The facilitation approach to the project was testing was multi-faceted. At the local level it explored how site-based novice IFs working together with novice external ACs could introduce a new piece of evidence. At an external facilitation level the project was gathering information on how novice ACs could manage this role and whether it was compatible with their primary teaching and research positions. And finally the project was evaluating the effectiveness of 'remote' external expert facilitation via a series of monthly teleconference calls between the Adelaide team and the ACs and their partner IFs.

Evaluation design

Two levels of evaluation were planned based on realist principles (Pawson and Tilley, 1997; Yin, 2009). The first was at the local level where teams supported by ACs and IFs undertook a KT project (single case). The second level (multiple cases combined into one overall analysis)

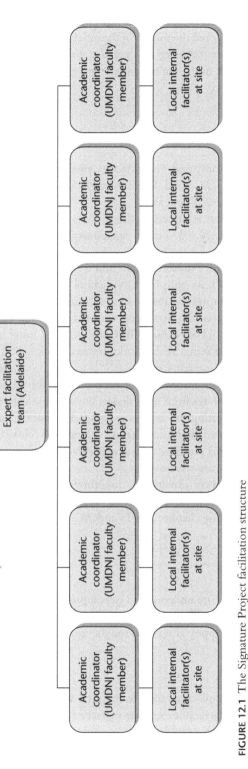

FIGURE 12.1 The Signature Project facilitation structure

involved the aggregation of the data from each clinical site together with the views and experiences of the facilitators about what worked and what did not. The expert facilitation research team explored the impact of the different facilitation roles on teams' ability to successfully introduce new evidence into practice, to understand and shape the local context and to engage individuals in the implementation process.

Method

Study participants comprised the following groups:

- Volunteer faculty and health facility personnel recruited to train as 'external academic coordinators' (ACs) and 'local internal facilitators' (IFs) for each of the six sites ($N = 1$ AC per site and 1–2 IFs per site).
- Team members recruited by the IFs to work with them on the implementation project (case) per site ($N = 3$–5 multi-disciplinary staff members per site).

The lead executive nurses in six healthcare facilities across New Jersey, with existing educational and clinical links with UMDNJ School of Nursing Faculty, were invited to participate in the Signature Project by the Dean of Nursing at UMDNJ.

Potential IFs from the sites along with potential ACs attended a three-day KT workshop hosted by the School of Nursing/JBI Collaborating Center in New Jersey and led by the University of Adelaide team. At the workshop an overview of the Signature Project was provided and expressions of interest sought.

The intervention process was interactive and involved the AC from the academic institution partnered with IFs from each clinical site working with clinicians in identifying a topic for improvement, locating the evidence, comparing current practice against the evidence-based practice recommendations, introducing strategies to 'close the gap' between the actual practice and the desired practice; re-evaluating the impact; and continuing this action cycle until improvements in care were evident.

IFs and ACs were involved in monthly teleconferences between the expert facilitator research project team and all the study sites. These teleconferences were used both as a support and learning mechanism for IFs and ACs as well as a data collection mechanism for the research team.

Ethics

Each participating site undertook to gain approval for their local projects with their own Institutional Review Boards (IRB). Participation in the Signature Project was conditional on IRB approval. Ethical approval was also sought and gained from both universities.

Data collection

A suite of data collection tools were used to gather baseline and follow-up data. These included data on facilitator experiences (facilitator checklists) plus ongoing self-report measures of process and progress; measures of context for each health facility using the Alberta Context Tool (ACT) (Estabrooks et al., 2009); an evidence utilisation checklist which provided ongoing recording of teams' reviews and use of evidence; and the completion of the PARIHS Self-Assessment Tool for leads and teams (Kitson et al., 2012).

In addition to these baseline and process measures, all facilitators shared their reflections and experiences at the monthly teleconferences in order to learn from each other's experiences.

Data analysis

Data sources included monthly teleconference transcripts, facilitator checklist data at the beginning of the project and interviews at the end, summaries of evidence meetings between facilitators and team members, data from the ACT and PARIHS self-report measures and, finally, audit data collected locally from each team with changes detected in their improvement plan.

Teleconference data were digitally recorded, transcribed and read by the evaluation team using the broad themes of evidence, context, individual and facilitation. Two members of the team read and re-read each transcript, identifying pieces of text that reflected an element of the main categories. These pieces of text were then aggregated into sub-themes and entered into NVIVO qualitative data analysis software.

Information about the local teams' understanding and use of evidence was gained from teleconference transcripts as well as individual support sessions and reflections from the academic coordinators. These data were also themed and sorted using NVIVO. The information on context was collated from the aforementioned data sources and supported using information from ACT. ACT data were aggregated to provide means and standard deviations for each site on each of the eight domains, namely leadership; culture; evaluation; social capital; formal interactions; informal interactions; structural and electronic resources; and organisational slack. Each site was then provided with a summary of this information along with comparisons of data from past research to provide an understanding of how the site compared to others (Schultz and Kitson, 2010).

Evaluating the impact of facilitation

The findings from the Signature Project will concentrate on the facilitation intervention and what we learnt about the different facilitation roles implemented and methods used to promote KT in these very different organisations. A short summary of how each site undertook its KT project will be presented, followed by an analysis and interpretation of how the facilitators experienced the process. Finally some thought will be given to what was learnt from the project and how it could be improved upon in future studies.

Characteristics of the sites

Site A summary

Site A was a small, 111-bed capacity community hospital in the north of the state, which provided a range of outpatient services ranging from cancer care through addiction counselling and diabetes care in addition to acute care services. This site became involved in the project because one of the IFs had previously studied at the university that provided the ACs. This hospital was actively looking for ways in which to incorporate research activities into their nursing practices and they felt that involvement in the project would benefit their organisation.

The workshop attendees (three senior nursing staff members) drew on recent Hospital Consumer Assessment of Healthcare Providers and Systems (HCAHPS) results to identify medication education as an area in which the hospital could improve its practice. Although not well resourced, this site began their facilitation journey with an established set of team members to run the project. The AC was allocated according to geographical proximity rather than expert knowledge of the intervention topic or familiarity with that particular hospital system. However, over the course of the project, national and state contextual changes led to the loss of a significant number of the initial project team.

The first hurdle this site experienced was obtaining IRB approval to be involved in the project. Unlike some of the other sites, site A did not have experience in obtaining IRB approval so the IFs and AC had to work very hard to explain what this was and why it was required. This led to a long delay to the commencement of the project that also coincided with the resignation of one of the original IFs. This IF was the clinical lead on the unit where the project was going to take place, which meant that the other two IFs (both senior managers) were impeded when trying to implement changes at the local level. Loss of connection to the ward lowered interest in the project. Furthermore, one of these IFs became ill and subsequently resigned from the hospital, leaving only one IF to run the project with the AC.

To make the situation even more volatile, the organisation itself then went through a major restructuring process that diverted the energy and focus of the IF away from the KT project and onto other aspects of their primary role and responsibilities. By this stage (several months into the project with little progress), the AC was feeling frustrated as they had not been able to forge a relationship with the staff in the hospital. Despite having some experience with facilitation projects in the past, the cumulative challenges presented by site A in terms of its volatile context and changing and relatively inexperienced IFs meant that the objective to improve medication education was not achieved.

However, in terms of overall reflections the views were that the experience had been more helpful than anticipated when considering the challenges they faced throughout the project. Ultimately though, some of the team members felt that the work was pointless in the face of major changes occurring in the broader health context:

> The original people (bar X) have all gone. There's also a lot of talk about the viability of the hospital . . . people have left and gone to another facility and a lot of operations facilities have left and gone to other private facilities. There have been significant changes in the external context that makes this initiative relatively insignificant in the scheme of things.
>
> *(AC site A)*

This reflection confirms the importance of the local and wider context and the timing of introducing new initiatives.

Site B summary

Site B, situated on the Atlantic Seaboard, was a 321-bed not-for-profit community hospital, which had Magnet designation, and was part of a large network of hospitals providing a range of health services across New Jersey. This hospital offered a range of inpatient and outpatient services, including advanced diagnostic, surgical and vascular services, the region's only Acute

Care for the Elderly unit, as well as a Primary Stroke Centre, Chest Pain Centre, Pharmacology Institute, and the state's first satellite emergency department.

This site became involved in the project because the lead IF had been working in evidence-based practice for several years and had a strong link with the Dean of the university facilitating the project. The intervention topic was determined through consultation with local health professionals, who were asked to highlight an area of particular interest to them. This hospital had a strong research culture and employed a range of staff who conducted research projects within the hospital as part of their capstone study requirements. Furthermore, this group was able to secure a grant to fund the involvement of one of the key clinical investigators and had access to research support personnel.

Site B was the most knowledgeable in terms of its understanding of evidence-based practice. The infrastructure to support evidence review and synthesis was good and both IFs were knowledgeable and expert in this part of their roles. An AC was allocated to site B at the beginning of the project but after a short period it was clear that the IFs were independent and did not require additional help. The prevailing context in the hospital was also supportive of ongoing professional development and innovation.

The topic site B selected was to implement the best available evidence in early delirium identification in elderly hip surgery patients. A review of the existing evidence was undertaken to find whether delirium predictor tools had been developed for this population group. The local team found no tools with a strong evidence base and so they developed and tested their own tool based upon evidence from their local context. They were supported in this activity by the nursing leadership, the research unit and they in turn were able to create a local environment where clinical nurses were mentored and supported. A quote from one of the IFs illustrates this:

> It was announced at our conference . . . at our nursing conference, the work that we're doing, so we have full administrative support . . . as far as trying to build some momentum for the project we created a mini steering committee. It was multidisciplinary from the get go and so that in turn made it such that all those members became champions for us in their respective locations.
>
> *(IF site B)*

The two IFs at site B were experienced researchers and it was clear from the data that they utilised their existing approach to evidence-based practice to undertake this project. The result of the first phase of the work was the development and testing of a delirium predictor tool for elderly fractured femur patients. Neither IF required nor desired support from either the research project team or the ACs. However, it is interesting to note that site B chose to undertake a piece of primary research (developing and testing a delirium predictor tool for elderly patients undergoing surgery) rather than select a piece of already existing evidence and track how it was implemented.

Site C summary

Site C was a large general medical and surgical facility providing a broad range of inpatient and outpatient services, including cancer services, bariatric services, a women's centre and geriatric services. The organisation was involved in the project initially because one of the clinical staff employed at the hospital was also a member of the faculty at UMDNJ. In order to identify the topic of the KT project the investigators chose a ward in the hospital and conducted an informal audit to identify a clinical issue. This audit identified that older patients at risk of deconditioning were not being provided with up-to-date activity orders and further to this were not being assisted to maintain physical condition. The clinical staff were able to secure a grant to support their research; they used this funding to employ several staff members to assist with project implementation (assisting patients to mobilise more) and data analysis. However, the project team found it difficult to secure multidisciplinary support for the project.

Site C had a partnership between the AC and the IF that was quite distinct from any of the other sites. The AC was a joint appointment between both organisations so she was not strictly an external facilitator. Neither the AC nor IF had been involved in such a project before and found the experience quite challenging. Although the AC had experience in research design and data collection she had not previously facilitated an implementation project. Several learning points were noted by both facilitators; first was the realisation that success was as much to do with negotiation and getting stakeholders on board as it was to do with achieving improvements in patient care. At one point the project ran into danger because of pushback from a multidisciplinary team member who felt they had not been properly involved in the process. The facilitators also struggled to implement change in a culture that was not particularly supportive of this type of initiative. Securing additional funding was one way in which this team was able to neutralise the issue.

The clinical team working with the facilitators to improve mobility and prevent deconditioning in patients during their hospital stay felt that they learnt a lot and really appreciated the support they had received. They were able to implement the suggestions into practice improvements and used this knowledge to shape new projects.

> It's like travelling through this unknown territory and you don't know what's going to come next. I don't know how to put it; you think you have it figured out. Like we thought we had the physical therapy on board and then the nursing assistants threw a curve ball. Well, okay, it's complicated and complex and there are a lot of players.
>
> *(AC site C)*

> [We] have devised an implementation study for the process based on this Signature experience . . . after they do the literature review for the project they will move forward with the KT protocol. We have followed the same model. So the whole approach seems to have worked and the committee are excited about this . . . I feel I have grown through this process. [I] have learnt a lot about the facilitator's role. I'm able to use it and transfer it into a different project with a different context.
>
> *(AC site C)*

Site D summary

Site D was a large, 600-bed, adult inpatient psychiatric facility providing a range of state-wide services: acute and chronic psychiatric care, geriatric psychiatric care, a sub-acute medical unit and a dual diagnostic unit for those with co-morbid developmental disabilities and mental health issues. This site became involved in the project because they had an IF who had recently picked up a role promoting evidence-based practice within the state-wide system and this person had established a close working relationship with one of the faculty members of the university who was externally facilitating the project. This faculty member brought the project to the attention of the IF, who was eager to participate as she felt that the project had the ability to benefit site D.

The project topic was an obvious choice for this hospital as a recent review had found that the overuse of PRN ('as needed') medication was an issue in the state. This facility was eager to address this issue by implementing an evidence-based practice activity. The whole-hospital system was perceived to be underfunded and as such there were few resources available to the project team. The project was led by a minimal number of staff and relied heavily on the assistance provided by the AC.

Site D also faced a number of senior staff changes during the time of the project: two of the three original IFs at the workshop retired or moved jobs, leaving one IF and the AC to manage the project. Despite this and the lack of resources the staff in site D became very engaged and interested in the project. Over the period of time that the team was addressing the PRN issue directly, other practices started to change; more activities were encouraged and more entertainment resources including TVs and stereos were introduced for patient use. This demonstrated an increase in the organisation's focus on the use of therapeutic interventions over medications for the management of patient behaviour.

The AC for site D was an experienced facilitator in her own right and it was very much through her commitment to and relationship with the senior nursing team in site D that members were able to achieve what they did. At the celebratory event marking the end of the project a large number of the hospital staff came to hear the presentation delivered regarding changes in their organisation and it was clear that the project had meant a lot for many staff.

> It got acknowledged at several of the hospital activities . . . by the CEO, so it was . . . they know that there was going to be something on that was different.
>
> *(AC site D)*

Site E summary

Site E was part of a large health group that provided home health, hospice and community-based services to over 120 000 people annually. This organisation was eager to form a relationship with the university to develop their research and quality improvement activities. This group identified their topic by researching the most common reasons for hospital re-admission in their patients. Given that the services they provided aimed to keep patients in their own home this was a key area for their organisation to explore. The audit identified cardiac issues as one of the most common reasons for hospital re-admission; from this the group consulted internally with local knowledge ambassadors and quality improvement staff to develop the project. Site E did not have a lot of research resources, the IF was one of the most knowledgeable in the organisation about how to conduct research but other staff members involved did not have this level of knowledge. However, the organisation was supportive of the project and a committee incorporating the aims of the project was formed during the study.

The IF for site E was replaced after the first few months of the project. It then became apparent that no one else in the organisation had been involved in the project. A second IF was appointed and a rapid update workshop was undertaken to get the wider team members up to speed. In addition a second AC joined the original AC who had been allocated to site E.

This second AC established a very positive working relationship with the newly appointed IF and together they started to move the project forward.

> And we're looking at just heart failure patients that went in for heart failure related admissions. So we really detailed the project down more and I met with [AC] and we looked at standards and then kind of pulled it all together . . . we have a new committee . . . it's called the homecare quality committee. So actually, that's going to start looking at acute care hospitalization rather than have all these other commit-tees . . . it's made up of some good leaders so that's alright . . . it's a good opportunity for [site D] – motivate them to do these sorts of projects. They want to do them, they just need support to get started.
>
> *(AC site E)*

Despite being a 'conscript' to the project, the AC settled into the work and was soon very much appreciated by the IF:

> I've met with [AC] a few times and she's really . . . enabled me to facilitate the project better and kind of kept me on track on what's going on. So she's been a great resource for myself and listening to what other people are saying. I'm really excited to continue to work with her and use her as a great resource.
>
> *(IF site E)*

One of the biggest challenges for both facilitators was working with staff who did not have a lot of research literacy. This meant that the facilitators had to continuously make the information easy to understand prompting a comment from the AC:

> I have learnt a lot about facilitation. It has been a satisfying experience – frustrating at the start but overall I consider it a positive experience and I would do it again.
>
> *(AC site E)*

Site F summary

Site F was a large tertiary care centre with 504 inpatient beds, accommodating up to 19,000 admissions annually and a further 215,000 outpatient visits. This hospital was linked to the university providing the external facilitation during the project and as such provided a natural partner to the project. However, staff from this site who were sent to the initial workshop were not aware of what the project would entail and therefore were not committed to following through with the necessary research activities. Furthermore, over the course of the project the relationship between the hospital and the UMDNJ began to change and this produced barriers to effective work.

The topic for the KT intervention was selected by the IFs at the initial workshop who per-ceived that infection control procedures around shared equipment were not being followed. The staff who attended the workshop were relatively junior registered nurses and shared an understandable anxiety that they would not be able to become IFs for such a project. The Dean of the Nursing School contacted the Executive Director for Nursing to clarify the purpose of the study and it was decided to continue with a different set of IFs.

There were limited resources available at site F for the project – staff who were interested in being involved in the project were not given any additional time to complete project-related tasks and very few of the staff at this site were experienced in conducting research. Furthermore, there was difficulty in securing the physical resources required for the project. The AC allocated to site F found it very difficult to arrange to meet with the IFs. Meetings were scheduled and cancelled repeatedly. When the AC and the IFs did find time to collaborate they organised a series of focus groups for registered nurses about the utilisation of shared non-critical patient equipment and how to reduce the risk of infection. To the AC's surprise the interest in the focus groups was considerable, indicating that the staff were more enthusiastic about the project than initially anticipated and may have lacked opportunities to become involved early on in the process. The project did not get further than the running of the focus groups before the timeframe for the project expired.

The AC summed up their experience:

> KT really takes a lot longer . . . two steps forward, three steps back. The [AC role] was really important to the environment that was not conducive to allowing time for development. If they had a QI [Quality Improvement] Coach who was part of the hospital that would have been better. Working at different levels of knowledge and facilitating is a great challenge . . . interpreting knowledge and evidence for different levels of staff to understand is a big challenge.
>
> *(AC site F)*

However, it is encouraging to note that the IF and AC together with their small team of registered nurses did eventually complete the project outside of the time period with resultant positive actions and experiences.

Facilitators' collective experiences

The following findings have emerged from the thematic analysis of the teleconference notes and the exit interviews with all the facilitators (both IFs and ACs) engaged in the project. From the original 13 IFs across the six sites, six were interviewed at the end of the projects. There was one IF from sites A, C, D and E; two from site B and none from site F. One AC per site was interviewed ($n = 6$) along with three additional faculty members (Project Leads, PL) who had been involved in the overall research project. Interviews were conducted via teleconference and ran for around 40–45 minutes each.

Even for those with experience, facilitating the Signature Project was a new and challenging experience. Both ACs and IFs would have liked more structure in terms of using the PARIHS framework. Some parts were familiar but others were less familiar and the language was different to what they had previously experienced. The facilitators were generally surprised by the lack of knowledge and skills around evidence-based practice and KT in the organisations and as a consequence the ACs in particular had to take on a much more active facilitation role than anticipated. Also, it was noted that much of the early engagement with the project was didactic and following instructions: if something is not in the required documentation then it does not get done.

Another major insight was the realisation from both the IFs and ACs that dealing with the complexity of context was one of the most important elements of the project. Successful facilitation involved knowing how to work the system. Most felt uncertain about what would happen after the project and there was a lack of confidence that what had been achieved would embed and start to grow within the system.

There was agreement from both the IFs and ACs about the need for more leadership in the local KT teams and more thought needed to be given to how more local team members could become involved in order to ensure there was sufficient capacity to create momentum and sustain interest. Difficulties at the local level were identified when ACs were not available to prompt project initiatives and this role was therefore seen to be useful in promoting change. Having someone slightly removed from the local context was seen as beneficial, especially in the early days when people were still unsure what they were supposed to be doing following the workshop.

The importance of collaborative relationships was emphasised, in particular for achieving successful implementation of new knowledge and for sustaining it. There was a view that the sense of success of a project was in large measure reliant on forming good relationships with teams at a local level. This was not easy to do and required a lot of work on the part of both the ACs and IFs. If these relationships were not formed at the beginning, then the project risked losing the goodwill and commitment of staff.

Facilitation was defined as the ability to achieve change without being directive or authoritative. This was important at an organisational level – where organisations had to be willing to be facilitated and able to define what they wanted from involvement. Another important feature of successful projects was that teams took the time to establish expectations early and ensured that there were systems in place to ensure that the teams committing to be involved in the project were held accountable for project aims. There was general agreement that closer links between universities and healthcare organisations would enable more effective facilitation and in the long run help build capacity and capability.

An essential characteristic of success was the involvement of appropriate key stakeholders at the local level. If they were not consulted and their opinions not respected, then it was an uphill battle. Progress was slow and the project risked stalling if there was no one committed or determined to keep it alive at that level. Furthermore, in many accounts there was a feeling of powerlessness amongst nurses to effect lasting change. Despite the range of roles held by those involved, such as quality and safety and research support, there still tended to be a disconnect from the lived experiences of nurses at the level of direct patient care. With a few notable exceptions, the general feeling was that the nursing voice was still weak in the system.

Reflections and lessons learnt

A total of 11 overarching themes were identified from the synthesis of the site case studies. Table 12.1 summarises these together with a preliminary attempt at constructing a hypothesis or proposition that could be further tested in future studies. Each theme will first be outlined:

1. The importance of collaborative relationships

Without collaboration by all stakeholders in each site successful KT was considered to be unlikely. These relationships needed to be established early in the project, preferably at its inception. The scope of the project had to be examined and all those potentially impacted needed to be consulted. These sentiments were illustrated by the following quotes:

> [AC] feels the whole thing (success) is about trust; knowing each other; building up that relationship and getting the feeling of trust that was building.
>
> *(AC site A)*

In particular, the importance of building trusting relationships was emphasised and the ability of the AC role in particular to have well-developed negotiating skills to achieve end results.

> Learning how to work with people without having authority over them and [being] able to get things done.
>
> *(AC site D)*

2. Getting buy-in from key stakeholders

> I didn't understand the politics and dynamics. I thought we had identified the key stake-holders from the very start but we didn't engage them to a level that we needed to until we were faced with the possibility of failure.
>
> *(AC site C)*

As mentioned above, this is crucial to KT success. Do not wait until barriers arise or the possibility of the project being successful is threatened. All stakeholders should have their input sought and considered throughout the KT project. The role of the ACs was particularly important in trying to manage the wider contextual issues as illustrated in the following quotes:

> We have not had a CNO; [we had an] Acting Director of Nursing. The CEO said 'Sure, go for it'. But the whole workforce is in a state of flux.
>
> *(IF site D)*

> This process required staff to volunteer to be involved so the facilitation process was more demanding or challenging – you had to get staff to actively engage and buy in to what you were doing. This did not happen easily at all. We kept talking about it, and finally at some point we reached a tipping point and threshold awareness was raised.
>
> *(AC and IF site C)*

3. Recognising the essential skills necessary for the successful progression of the project

Successful facilitation requires a range skills including but not limited to project management, negotiation, moderation, motivation and awareness. Facilitators need to have or receive training in these skills. The relationship between the ACs and the IFs was seen as positive in terms of mutual support and development:

> [IF site E] was very receptive to the learning process. She was leading the team and getting the others to participate.
>
> *(AC site E)*

Equally, this recognition was identified by the IFs as well:

> My bosses in EBP [evidence-based practice] were all for it so that's how I tried to work. I was fortunate to have [AC site D] as a mentor and colleague as not many people in the system had the requisite knowledge.
>
> *(IF site D)*

4. Measure success via practice change, improvements in context and personal relationships

The sum of a facilitation project should not only be calculated by achievement of the new practice. The broader ramifications of the project, including improved inter-professional collaboration, site receptiveness to change and the professional development of those involved should not be overlooked. As the following quote reflects, the sites all started at different points in their learning journeys and so the job of the facilitators was very much to tailor the new knowledge to the context within which they found themselves. For some this was more challenging than others:

> All is not lost, we are moving along and trying to get it done . . . next week (training) . . . we're moving from one step to the next. God knows this organisation needs it!
>
> *(AC site F)*

> [I] can see that the effect of the Signature Project is spreading to other parts of the geriatric group in the hospital. The hospital has an initiative on mobility . . . where it is identifying champions and starting to review journal articles. [It] means that the learning from Signature can influence this process.
>
> *(IF site C)*

5. Feeling like an outsider

Facilitators need support and encouragement. It can be an isolating experience. However being viewed as an objective participant in the KT process can be beneficial and it can break down barriers between and within professions and clinical areas. For external facilitators in particular it is important to know how to manage that feeling of being an outsider with little influence:

> The first challenge I had was that I did not have a relationship with the people at the hospital. I had not experienced such a situation where I was attempting to do research without some sort of prior relationship. I felt this was not as effective as previous encounters.
>
> *(AC site A)*

This feeling of exclusion was mediated by the relationship between the AC and the IF. When managed effectively it had the potential to be very powerful:

> Initially, staff's reaction to [AC site C] was 'Who's she?' Always go back to the research project – something new and then I could 'blame' [AC] for getting us involved! It was

a good tactic and it worked. [AC] would be introduced as the nurse researcher, she was the change agent from outside.

(IF site C)

6. Using past experience to shape facilitation

Although the terminology relating to facilitation and KT may have been unfamiliar to some, the skills and tools to achieve this are often linked to other experiences. The IFs in site B, for example, had extensive experience in evidence-based practice and they drew on this to shape the beginning of the project:

> Lead people through evidence; let them look at the articles, doing searches, and guiding them. It involves IT, policy change, education, and communication. We both have links to several different universities, which helps build sustainability and capacity. Students from every level, from associate degrees to PhDs.
>
> *(IF1&2 site B)*

Drawing on past experiences also enabled facilitators to reflect upon their own learning journey in terms of the PARIHS framework and the KT Toolkit:

> Intuitively (I) felt that the framework 'fitted' or made sense. I knew where I was going but I did not have a deep understanding . . . before I never really got these intricacies down.
>
> *(AC site D)*

7. Importance of structure, direction and understanding from the start

All those involved in a KT project must have a clear understanding of the processes and expected outcomes. Breaking this information up into 'bite size chunks' is a useful strategy to assist in this process. The feedback from the interviews indicated that the initial workshop tried to cover too much information in too fast a time and that participants did not really understand the full implications of the project:

> There was too much in the initial three days and people did not remember the detail, especially the practice sites. How can we break up the learning giving the participants 'bite size chunks' of learning that will make sense and they will remember, especially the practice areas.
>
> *(PL)*

This is an important observation as it required the expert facilitation team to consider how best to present the content of the KT Toolkit.

8. Clarity around the level of commitment

Facilitation of KT takes time and employers and team members must consider this. Expectations to achieve KT within current workloads are, for many, unrealistic. Acknowledgement of the commitment and time required demonstrates the project is valued and supported by the organisation. In addition, the facilitation role can expose deficits in knowledge and skills, which need to be addressed in a respectful and proactive way to optimise the success of the project:

> What is surprising is that the ACs are less prepared for this facilitative role than anticipated. No one was prepared for the lack of knowledge, resources or skills in the organisations. This meant the AC role became much more directive and active than was anticipated and it took everyone by surprise.
>
> *(PL)*

9. Importance of the AC role

The external AC team were seen to assist in several ways. First, they contributed through the provision of resources such as education, tools and assistance with evaluation. Second, their ability to comment objectively on project aims, progress and goals was valued. Third, the ACs set and maintained the timeframe for the projects, thus giving them overall structure and an imperative to deliver at certain milestones within each site. The other contribution of the ACs was to bring together a range of skills and attributes from research, education and quality improvement into a 'package' that was focused on implementation:

> Other nurse researchers don't know how to incorporate research into practice. Educators need to be taught those skills too. We need to stop 'throwing' information at people and start working with them to help them implement it.
>
> *(AC site C)*

10. Receptivity of context

An assessment of the context prior to commencement of KT was seen as essential. Identification of strengths and barriers in this area helped to identify stakeholders and plan interventions. Yet, it was clear that even the best attempts of the facilitators were not sufficiently potent to counteract stronger prevailing contextual factors:

> Cultural context is so paramount to everything else. Cognitive aspect, knew what to do but what was difficult was the process of putting it all in place, like a game. Have to be very strategic . . . no nursing administrative support, no communication. Nursing Admin not interested.
>
> *(AC site F)*

11. The KT Toolkit in the future

The practical tools provided in the toolkit assisted in participants' understanding of the impact and evaluation of context, evidence and facilitation. The influence of the individual and how this could be evaluated and was seen as a potentially valuable addition to the existing toolkit. Equally, participants' utilisation of the toolkit and experiences of the facilitation approaches have helped to add to the growing body of knowledge in this complex area:

What I appreciated from the project was the experience of combining a whole systems approach to change with the practical tools and techniques of facilitating small groups, undertaking QI type initiatives and helping teams understand about evidence.

(AC site D)

What this case study adds to our overall understanding of facilitation

In conducting a facilitation project the preparatory phase must not be underestimated. All involved must be clear about what is occurring and what their roles and responsibilities are. It is most important to establish the knowledge and capabilities of those who will be directly

TABLE 12.1 Summary of themes emerging from case study data

Key themes from facilitator interviews and other sources	Emerging propositions to be tested
1. The importance of collaborative relationships	Collaboration across and between different stakeholder groups is essential for successful KT activity
2. Getting buy-in from key stakeholders	Methods to enable different groups to commit to a shared goal is essential for successful KT activity
3. Recognising the essential skills necessary for the successful progression of the project	Facilitators need to be carefully selected against clearly defined, evidence-based criteria
4. Measuring success via practice change, improvements in context and personal relationships	Success criteria need to be developed in three broad dimensions: practice change (linked to the innovation); improvements in contextual dimensions; and improvements in personal attitudes, behaviours, and working practices
5. Feeling like an outsider	A primary goal for the external facilitator is to manage the feeling of being treated as an outsider
6. Using past experience to shape facilitation	Facilitators need to be reflective practitioners, building on past experiences to shape current and future learning
7. Importance of structure, direction and understanding from the start	Structured learning in a staged way is important to the success of the KT project
8. Clarity around the level of commitment	It is important to be clear about the investment required by the project. Investment links to an assessment of capacity around context, innovation and the individual
9. Importance of the external facilitator role	External facilitators need to be more explicit about what they can and cannot achieve
10. Receptivity of context	Context is central to success. It is vital that facilitators understand this and have a range of tools and techniques to diagnose and create interventions that will address the challenges
11. The KT Toolkit in the future	The KT Toolkit needs to be continuously reviewed in order to optimise its impact

involved with clinicians to be able to effectively provide them with what they will need for the project. Although previous projects have begun with a similar type of workshop to 'set the scene', for this project it was apparent that those attending had quite different levels of understanding about KT generally and specifically what would be required of them. Some had considerable knowledge and experience but for others this type of activity was completely new. Some of the organisations involved were very well resourced while others were resource poor. Many other contextual issues impacted on the project.

The dual purpose of the project was difficult for many of the organisations to come to grips with. The work being done at the local level in each organisation was easy to understand: the teams examining an issue of concern with the aim of improving patient care using the best evidence. What was more difficult was understanding the role of the ACs in researching the process and creating new knowledge about facilitation. The IRBs were mostly not familiar with this type of research and were wary about data leaving their organisation and being used by 'outsiders'. Managing this lack of understanding caused considerable delays.

Another question that was explored through this study was how well the PARIHS framework could assist in understanding what was happening at each of the sites. In regard to evidence for many of the projects there was reasonably sound objective evidence to inform practice. Each of the teams was assisted to identify appropriate evidence to inform practice and to then use the evidence to develop auditing tools to measure their practice. The exception was site B who had difficulty in identifying good evidence to support practice. They then embarked upon a primary research project to develop the evidence they needed to guide their practice. This necessarily delayed the translation component of the project significantly. This speaks to the motivation of KT projects. If the trigger for a KT project is the emergence of new evidence then the evidence is there to support practice change. If the impetus for the KT project is poor performance or even a sentinel event there is not always going to be good external evidence available and as a result the project may struggle. Although it is strategic to focus on projects where there is good external evidence available, there will be occasions where the imperative to deal with a problem is greater than the lack of evidence.

In considering context it was very apparent that this remains a defining element of success in changing practice. At the initial workshop participants were asked to consider aspects of context within their organisations. In hindsight this examination of context was not sufficient to inform the facilitation process. In time the local facilitators would come to better understand the complex contextual issues that impacted on their projects but this was not the case during the initial workshop. In some previous projects the expert facilitators were more familiar with the clinical settings where the projects were to occur and the contextual issues were more apparent. Again adjustments to the preparatory phase would likely have assisted here. There were, however, many examples of contextual issues that were overcome in time. Site D, for instance, was disadvantaged by a lack of resources and systems to monitor and improve practice. The AC and IF worked hard to engage those directly involved in the project but also the staff in the wider organisation. The wide support for the project was very evident at the celebration event at the end of the project.

One emerging theme to come from this project was that of the 'individual'. The PARIHS framework very much considers evidence, context and facilitation at an organisation level. However, organisations are made up of individuals and there were several sites where quite distinctly the actions and impact of individuals required closer scrutiny. Site E had to replace their IF some time after commencement of the project. This would normally have been a significant blow to the project but the drive and willingness of the new recruit quickly made up for lost time. Site C also ran into an individual who felt they had been unduly left out of the project and became very obstructive. Undeterred, the AC and IF understood the crucial need to bring this person into the project, albeit belatedly.

What was also different about this project was the remote nature of the expert facilitators from Australia. Although the initial workshop was face-to-face, throughout the project monthly meetings and additional support sessions were conducted by phone. Although all agreed the monthly meetings were useful and the external and peer support valuable, there was a sense of the facilitation not being as direct and as tailored as it should have been. In other projects the expert facilitators have worked more closely with the clinicians. The use of the ACs in this project was supposed to bridge the gap between the expert facilitators and those working on the ground, but the ACs also needed support.

Concluding comments

In judging the overall success of the project there are a number of elements to consider. First, the context was extremely difficult. Many of the organisations involved were in an extreme period of change. There were economic pressures on most of the organisations that made resourcing of the projects difficult. Many of those involved were not familiar with KT and had a very steep learning curve. There were many personal aspects that impacted on the ACs and IFs. There were illnesses, retirements and pregnancies, resulting in key personnel moving in and out of projects at unexpected times. Despite this there were many signs of success. There was clearly a greater level of understanding and respect between academic and clinical colleagues. All involved had a much better understanding of KT, even the IRBs. There was a great sense of wanting to build on and continue the work. At least three publications were produced by teams of IFs and ACs from the individual projects (Bugel and Scuderi, 2013; Russell-Babin and Miley, 2013; Holly et al., 2014). Some of the teams had not achieved measurable changes to practice or patient outcomes by the formal end of the project but there was a determination to keep going to achieve that change, as was noted for site F.

And finally, what can organisations such as JBI collaborating centres learn from this experience and how can KT implementation toolkits be tested in the future? Our collective experiences would suggest the following: plan carefully; select participating organisations that have the resource, commitment and infrastructure to support the initiative; prepare the IFs and ACs more thoroughly at the beginning; set realistic timeframes; and above all keep the communication open and constructive, particularly when time and distance separate the two collaborating teams.

References

Bugel, M.J. & Scuderi, D. 2013. Addressing the use of shared medical equipment in a large urban hospital. In: Holly, C. (ed.) *Scholarly Inquiry*. New York: Springer.

Estabrooks, C., Squires, J., Cummings, G., Birdsell, J. & Norton, P. 2009. Development and assessment of the Alberta Context Tool. *BMC Health Services Research*, 9, 234.

Holly, C., Percy, M., Caldwell, B., Echevarria, M., Bugel, M.J. & Salmond, S. 2014. Moving evidence to practice: reflections on a multisite academic-practice partnership. *International Journal of Evidence Based Healthcare*, 12, 31–8.

Kitson, A., Harvey, G. & McCormack, B. 1998. Enabling the implementation of evidence based practice: a conceptual framework. *Quality in Health Care*, 7, 149–59.

Kitson, A., Rycroft-Malone, J., Harvey, G., McCormack, B., Seers, K. & Titchen, A. 2008. Evaluating the successful implementation of evidence into practice using the PARIHS framework: theoretical and practical challenges (2008). *Implementation Science*, 3, 1.

Kitson, A., Wiechula, R., Salmond, S. & Jordan, Z. 2012. *Knowledge Translation in Healthcare*. Philadelphia, PA: Lippincott Williams and Wilkins.

Pawson, R. & Tilley, N. 1997. *Realistic Evaluation*. Thousand Oaks, CA: Sage.

Pearson, A., Wiechula, R., Court, A. & Lockwood, C. 2005. The JBI model of evidence-based healthcare. *International Journal of Evidence-Based Healthcare*, 3, 207–15.

Russell-Babin, K.A. & Miley, H. 2013. Implementing the best available evidence in early delirium identification in elderly hip surgery patients. *International Journal of Evidence-Based Healthcare*, 11, 39–45.

Schultz, T. & Kitson, A. 2010. Measuring the context of care in an Australian acute care hospital: a nurse survey. *Implementation Science*, 5, 60.

Stetler, C., Legro, M., Rycroft-Malone, J., Bowman, C., Curran, G., Guihan, M., et al. 2006. Role of 'external facilitation' in implementation of research findings: a qualitative evaluation of facilitation experiences in the Veterans Health Administration. *Implementation Science*, 1, 23.

Wiechula, R., Kitson, A., Marcoionni, D., Page, T., Zeitz, K. & Silverston, H. 2009. Improving the fundamentals of care for older people in the acute hospital setting: facilitating practice improvement using a knowledge translation (KT) tool kit. *International Journal of Evidence-Based Healthcare*, 7, 283–95.

Yin, R.K. 2009. *Case Study Research: Design and Methods*. Thousand Oaks, CA: Sage.

13

MOVING FORWARD ON THE FACILITATION JOURNEY

Gill Harvey and Alison Kitson

Introduction

In this the final chapter of the book, our aim is to pull together the material from the previous chapters and set out what we think the next steps are. We begin by collating the key lessons from the five case studies that have been presented in Chapters 8–12. This includes comparing the similarities and differences across the cases, in order to identify useful insights into the facilitator role and the facilitation process within different contextual settings. We will also reflect on what the case study experiences tell us in relation to the revised i-PARIHS (integrated Promoting Action on Research Implementation in Health Services) framework and the facilitation model that we have presented in this book. Finally, we will address the question of 'what happens next'. For readers of the book, this will include thinking about where you are starting in terms of your own facilitation journey, whether as novice facilitators about to facilitate a new implementation project, or more experienced facilitators wanting to develop your knowledge and skills further and prepare others to take on the facilitator role. From our own perspective, we will reflect on our journey in writing this book and what we think the future challenges are in terms of ongoing research and development into implementation and facilitation in healthcare.

Comparing across the case studies

In the previous chapters, we have presented five case studies applying facilitator roles and facilitation methods in different settings, on different topics and with different combinations of internal-external and novice-experienced-expert facilitators. Chapter 8 described a project in the UK with novice facilitators, supported by an expert facilitation team, working within an improvement collaborative model to address the identification and management of chronic kidney disease in primary care. In Chapter 9, we presented a European study involving novice facilitators in four different countries and supported virtually by expert external facilitators to implement evidence-based recommendations for improving continence care in nursing home settings. The implementation setting for Chapter 10 was Vietnam, where novice external facilitators, with support from more experienced external facilitators, worked with local community groups to improve neonatal care. Chapter 11 focused on a project in an acute hospital setting in Australia, where experienced internal facilitators, working in partnership with external expert facilitators, supported a hospital-wide initiative to improve nutritional care of older adults in hospital. Finally in Chapter 12, we presented a facilitation study which brought together two Joanna Briggs Collaborating Centres (http://joannabriggs.org/JBC.aspx), one from the United States and the other from Australia. Here expert facilitators from one centre prepared and then virtually supported novice and experienced facilitators in the other centre to introduce evidence-based changes in six different organisations.

So what can we learn from these diverse case studies that involved facilitators working in seven different countries, on a total of ten different topics, across a range of acute, primary care, mental health and community settings. Table 13.1 provides a comparative overview of the five cases in terms of the facilitator roles and facilitation methods that were employed. These are discussed in some more detail in the following sections.

Facilitator roles in the case studies

The majority of the cases used novice facilitators in a mix of internal and external roles. The exception to this was the nutrition in older adults' project (Chapter 11) that started with experienced facilitators, who then recruited local champions to work with them. The facilitators mostly came from clinical backgrounds, although the chronic kidney disease (CKD) case had a mix of non-clinical and clinical novice facilitators and the neonatal case recruited lay people as novice facilitators. Individuals came into the facilitator roles by different routes: some were volunteers, some were nominated by their managers and others were formally recruited. In all cases, the novice and experienced facilitators were supported and mentored by expert external facilitators, some via close working, face-to-face relationships and other by more distant, virtual arrangements.

Preparation for commencing in the facilitator role also varied. In the neonatal study and the projects working with virtual external facilitator support, a formal training programme was held at the start of the project. However, in the CKD case, where the novice facilitators were part of a wider facilitation team, and in the nutrition project which started with more experienced facilitators, learning and development took place in a more continuous and incremental way. Across the cases, it was apparent that the novice facilitators grew in confidence as their skills, knowledge and experience in the facilitator role developed. However, the extent of their learning and development was related to a number of factors, including their position within the organisation where they were facilitating and their perceived level of influence, the peer support they experienced and the wider support from leaders and senior managers.

Facilitation methods and approaches

All five cases underpinned the design of their project with the PARIHS framework. This was generally used as an heuristic to frame the projects in terms of a focus on evidence, context and facilitation. In relation to evidence, the cases demonstrated different entry points. Some started with a pre-identified topic, for which there was existing evidence about best practice and collectively agreed aims for implementation based on the evidence. Others had an overall objective, for example, to reduce neonatal mortality, but allowed local teams to decide what aspect

TABLE 13.1 Comparing facilitator roles and facilitation methods across the five case studies

	Improving the identification and management of CKD in primary care (England)	Improving continence care for older adults in nursing homes (England, Ireland, Netherlands, Sweden)	Reducing neonatal mortality in rural communities (Vietnam)	Improving nutritional care of older adults in hospital (Australia)	6 locally determined topics: • Medication education in community hospitals • Early identification of delirium in older patients undergoing hip surgery • Maintaining physical activity in older adults in hospital • Reducing overuse of PRN medication in a mental health hospital setting • Reducing cardiac re-admissions to hospital • Infection control (USA)
Topic and setting					
Facilitator roles	Novice external and internal facilitators, supported by multi-professional facilitation team, including expert facilitator, clinical leader, project manager and information analyst Novice facilitators selected via an assessment panel and interview Embedded learning and development programme for novice facilitators	Novice internal facilitators virtually supported by external expert facilitators Novice facilitators identified by managers, according to criteria for role specification Initial 3-day training programme	Novice external facilitators supported by experienced and expert external facilitators Facilitators recruited from the Women's Union Attended a 2-week training programme	Experienced, volunteer internal facilitators, supported by external expert facilitators Internal facilitators recruited 'local champions' to work with them Minimal training required due to prior experience	Volunteer novice internal and external facilitators virtually supported by external expert facilitators Initial 3-day training workshop for novice facilitators

(continued)

TABLE 13.1 (continued)

Facilitation methods and approach	Underpinned by PARIHS framework	Underpinned by PARIHS framework	Underpinned by PARIHS framework	Underpinned by PARIHS framework	Implementation of a structured KT kit, derived from PARIHS
	Improvement collaborative model (learning events, monthly action periods, monthly audit and feedback)	Goal-focused approach, incorporating agreed aims, audit and feedback	Use of PDSA cycles to identify, prioritise and respond to local problems	Focus on the introduction of 3 evidence-based interventions	Each site selected their own topic for implementation
	Regular practice visits by facilitators	Monthly teleconference meetings between internal and external facilitators	Monthly supervision meetings between novice facilitators and external expert facilitators	Pre and post-implementation audit, plus further end of project audit	Monthly teleconference calls between expert and novice facilitators
	Monthly meetings of the facilitation project team	Internal evaluation, plus part of an RCT with process and outcome evaluation	RCT evaluation	Monthly meetings between external and internal facilitators	Comparative case study evaluation, within and across cases
	Internal, formative evaluation			Evaluation via audit data and stepped wedge RCT	

Abbreviations: CKD, chronic kidney disease; PARIHS, Promoting Action on Research Implementation in Health Services; PDSA, Plan–Do–Study–Act; RCT, randomised controlled trial; KT, knowledge translation.

of the overall topic they wanted to focus on. In other cases, such as the US Signature Project, local teams had freedom to identify the issue they wanted to work on. For some, this involved generating evidence to inform practice, especially in the absence of an existing evidence base.

In terms of facilitation strategies that were applied to address the project aims or objectives, all the cases used improvement methods and approaches, for example, Plan–Do–Study–Act (PDSA) cycles or audit and feedback, either individually or in combination. In keeping with recognised improvement methodology, the facilitators identified improvement teams to work with at a local level and provided ongoing support, for example, through regular meetings and visits, to apply the improvement methods in practice. For some novice facilitators, this presented a significant challenge, as was the case in the continence project where the novice facilitators were trying to develop their own knowledge and skills in audit at the same as supporting their colleagues to implement new practices.

The way in which the local facilitators addressed contextual issues varied across the cases, partly because they faced different contextual challenges, some at a health system level and others at an organisational, departmental or team level. In some cases, a formal context assessment was undertaken, usually at the start of the project, using either an established or locally developed tool. In other cases, survey methods and focus group discussions were held to review the local context and identify potential barriers to implementation. Ongoing review of contextual barriers – and discussion of appropriate facilitation strategies to deal with these – took place in most of the projects, particularly at the meetings between expert and more novice facilitators. In terms of the wider context, a mix of both formal and informal stakeholder engagement and involvement strategies was apparent. The more formalised approaches typically involved identifying clear support from senior managers and leaders and agreeing a communication strategy to keep key stakeholders informed about the project.

Evaluation strategies also varied across the cases and included a mix of both formative and summative approaches. In most cases, the facilitators were part of a formal implementation research study, where process and outcome data were collected to evaluate the impact of the facilitation intervention. However, formative evaluation also took place to enable ongoing review of progress, typically using locally collected data. This provided a useful way for the facilitators to track how the projects were going, to provide positive feedback to local teams or identify problems or barriers that were getting in the way.

Lessons learnt across the case studies

Reflecting on the lessons learnt within the case study chapters, a number of common themes emerge. These are summarised in Box 13.1. Overall, the cases illustrate that it is possible for novice facilitators to support implementation projects, provided they have support and mentorship from more experienced facilitators. This can be provided by face-to-face contact with expert facilitators or via virtual support methods; however, the experiences reported in the case studies would suggest that there are some limitations with virtually provided expert facilitation. For future projects employing virtual support by expert facilitators, it might be better to supplement the virtual methods with some more direct contact between expert and novice facilitators. In some cases novice and experienced facilitators worked in pairs, which appeared to offer benefits in terms of peer support.

BOX 13.1 LESSONS LEARNED ACROSS THE CASE STUDIES

- Importance of good project management:

    - Aims
    - Preparatory phase
    - Deadlines
    - Breaking the project down into manageable 'chunks'

- Need to balance structured approach with flexibility
- Importance of building relationships
- Being realistic in terms of aims and expectations; allowing enough time to see impact
- Need for leadership support and championing
- Can have different starting points within projects e.g. can start from existing evidence or from a local problem/priority
- Defining influence of context on implementation
- Need to pay attention to the people involved in and affected by implementation (e.g. chair of the group, unit leader, senior clinicians and staff who are not in the immediate improvement or implementation team)
- Need to pay attention to selection and preparation of facilitators
- Can have different combinations of facilitators, but possible to identify some guiding principles:

    - Importance of peer and expert support
    - Need for content and process expertise
    - Benefits of face-to-face contact between novice and expert facilitators

- Importance of planning for sustainability

Achieving a balance between structuring the project to achieve agreed aims and goals whilst at the same time retaining the flexibility to deal with contextual and process factors emerges as a critical skill for facilitators. This requires someone in the facilitator role who has sound judgement alongside organisational skills and who is able to cope with a degree of uncertainty and adapt to the unexpected. Good project management appears important to keep the project manageable from the both the facilitator's and the recipients' perspective. This involves undertaking the necessary preparation before the start of the project, agreeing clear aims and establishing appropriate deadlines. However, this project management role has to be undertaken in a sensitive and non-rigid way, with a constant eye on individual, team or contextual issues at a local level that may be presenting barriers to progress. In part, this depends upon the facilitator having spent time to understand the local context and build the necessary relationships at the outset of the project. It also involves paying attention to the wider stakeholders whose support and encouragement is needed to achieve the desired goals. In several of the cases, the need for a strong, clear relationship between the facilitator and local leaders was evident.

Projects can start from different points in terms of implementation depending on the particular circumstances at a local level, for example, identified needs and priorities, local champions and availability of evidence. Those projects where there is an underlying evidence base on which to design, plan and agree project aims and measures appear to make quicker progress.

However, progress is often slower than initially anticipated due to a combination of factors, including the facilitator's skills and confidence, local and organisational barriers or wider system-level factors.

Contextual factors feature strongly within the case study data, in terms of determining the way in which implementation projects take shape and progress. They can pose particular challenges for novice facilitators who are trying to get to grips with the role; direct contact and support from more experienced facilitators is particularly important here. This raises a number of issues, such as: having the right support and development structure for novice facilitators; creating ways for facilitators to support each other through peer contact and networks; and paying careful attention to the initial selection and preparation of facilitators.

It is clear from the five cases studied that there is no single 'right way' to facilitate an implementation project, however there are helpful pointers to follow and equally other things to avoid. Starting off the facilitation journey with attention to these issues should also help to ensure that innovation and improvement can be sustained over the longer term.

Reflections on the case studies in relation to the i-PARIHS framework and the facilitation model

We turn now to consider what the case study experiences tell us in relation to the revised i-PARIHS framework and the facilitation model that we presented in earlier chapters of the book. In Chapter 3 we proposed a re-conceptualisation of PARIHS, based on an integration of experiential and empirical evidence from users of the framework with relevant theoretical literature. This integrated PARIHS framework (i-PARIHS) proposed that successful implementation results from the facilitation of an innovation with the recipients in their context. We then presented a facilitation model that could be used to operationalise i-PARIHS. This was based on the idea of individuals working in facilitator roles (novice, experienced and expert) using facilitation strategies and methods to enable implementation, taking account of innovation, recipient and inner and outer contextual factors.

The case study data that we have just analysed and compared provides us further empirical evidence upon which to check out the propositions that we made within i-PARIHS and the associated facilitation model. We intend to do this by addressing the following questions:

- Is 'innovation' a more appropriate focus than 'evidence' when looking at 'what' is being implemented?
- Are the recipients of implementation an important group to consider separately from the innovation and the context?
- Is it helpful to separate out the different elements of inner and outer context?
- Is facilitation the element that can actively coordinate and enable the other three constructs? And if so:
  - is a goal-focused approach, working from the innovation outwards, a useful way to frame implementation projects in practice?
  - what skills and knowledge do facilitators need to practice the role within implementation projects?
- What are the important areas for ongoing research and development?

Adopting an innovation focus

In the i-PARIHS framework we have suggested a shift from focusing on 'evidence' to 'innovation' when thinking about and facilitating implementation. As we explained in Chapter 3, this is because the concept of innovation recognises the fluid way in which new ideas take shape as they are developed and introduced, in part because of the interaction between the innovation, the intended users and their specific situation. Innovation also embraces wider perceptions of evidence to inform practice, including both explicit and tacit knowledge, and innovation theory recognises that processes of experiential and situated learning shape the innovation journey. This aligns with the underlying philosophy of our general approach to implementation and facilitation. It also fits with the way in which implementation projects appear to evolve and progress in healthcare, often starting from different points in relation to underlying sources of knowledge, as the case studies illustrate.

What is also apparent from the case studies is the degree of overlap between the concepts of evidence-based practice, knowledge translation, innovation, improvement and implementation. Although from a research perspective, there are often distinctions made, for example, between improvement and implementation science, in practice there is a great deal more convergence. Implementation or knowledge translation projects are fundamentally concerned with improving the organisation and delivery of health services and patient care. As such, they commonly apply the principles and methods of quality improvement to structure and guide the process of introducing and evaluating changes in practice. The core elements of improvement methodologies (for example, establishing goals for improvement, agreeing and applying measures to evaluate progress and using small-scale testing to introduce and review changes) provide a helpful way of structuring an implementation project. However, as the case studies have illustrated, there is typically a discrete step at the start of the implementation project that involves establishing an evidence base to underpin the project, whether that is in the form of existing research evidence or involves the collation and synthesis of local evidence.

In conclusion, the concept of innovation – defined as anything perceived as new by the intended user – appears a useful way to describe the focus of implementation. However, this requires closer attention to the evidence base which underpins the innovation process, checking out that the proposed changes reflect current thinking about 'best practice'. This involves applying evidence from research, from clinical and patient observations and experiences, and from other data collected at a local and national level. Perhaps in future we should be talking about applying evidence-based innovation as a first step towards bringing together worldviews around innovation, improvement and implementation in healthcare.

Recipients as a discrete group for consideration

We have proposed the recipients – that is, the individual and collective audiences for the innovation – as a new construct within the i-PARIHS framework. The theoretical and empirical data strongly support this addition, although it is important to recognise that the recipients cannot be considered in isolation from the innovation or their context. It is very clear from the case studies that the facilitators and the implementation/improvement teams they work with often have to convince their colleagues that the proposed innovation is worthwhile in order to secure their commitment to making the required changes. In the CKD project (Chapter 8), there was an issue convincing some general practitioners that CKD was a real disease state that needed to be addressed and improved – an example of how the evidence–innovation–individual recipient relationship can play out. In the continence project (Chapter 9), there was the challenge of shifting mind-sets within many of the caregivers who had traditionally seen incontinence as the natural state in frail older residents. Here the issue was one around recipients' beliefs at a collective team level.

Relationships between the various people involved in leading, facilitating and supporting implementation also have an obvious impact on the processes and outcomes of the project. In some cases, this involves the interaction between the facilitator and the colleagues they are working with, including whether the facilitator is perceived to be credible in the role. At other times it can be about the relationship between the facilitator and the group leader or chair, or between the facilitator and formal and informal leaders at a local or organisational level. Consequently, the facilitator needs to be aware of the myriad of individual and collective factors that can impact upon implementation. For these reasons, we think that the recipient construct – encompassing both individual and collective motivation and ability to change – is a helpful additional construct within the i-PARIHS framework.

Widening the notion of context

A third area where we proposed a revision to the original PARIHS framework was to widen out the notion of context to incorporate the immediate local context, the wider organisational context and the external or outer context. With in the case studies, we have seen examples where these different levels of context exert an influence. For example, at the immediate level of implementation, the prevailing organisational culture may be resistant to change or to the particular new ideas presented by the innovation, as was the case with the continence project amongst many of the nursing home staff (Chapter 9). At the organisational level, issues such as re-organisation and re-structuring typically presented barriers to implementation, creating a period of instability, shifting the priorities within organisations or bringing in new senior leaders and managers with different values and beliefs. The disruptive influence of organisational factors such as these was evident in several of the case studies, including the individual implementation projects within the Signature Project (Chapter 12). Finally, things happening in the external health system also had a knock-on effect on implementation at a local level. The continence project provided examples of this: for example, the focus on continence within external regulatory inspection provided a driver for innovation and change at a practice level; conversely, the fact that specialist nurses employed by incontinence product companies provided much of the education on continence in the nursing home sector acted as a barrier. These examples provide some support for separating out the levels of context that need to be addressed during the process of implementation.

There is also evidence within the case studies that with the right facilitation and with sufficient time, it is possible to overcome contextual barriers. The neonatal study (Chapter 10) illustrates this clearly. Although working with lay facilitators in a health system that was hierarchically structured and managed, significant improvements in neonatal mortality were observed in the third year of the study. This highlights the potential contribution that facilitation can make, given the right people are in the facilitator roles, with a supportive infrastructure and sufficient time and resource to facilitate the required changes. Conversely, novice facilitators without the right level of skills, knowledge or influence, or lacking in guidance and support from a more experienced mentor, can find the contextual challenges encountered quite daunting. We turn now to look more specifically at the facilitation process and facilitator roles.

Facilitation as the 'active ingredient' of implementation

The final revision within the i-PARIHS framework is to explicitly position facilitation as the active ingredient that integrates action around the innovation and the recipients within their local, organisational and wider health system context to enable effective implementation. Facilitation in this respect refers to individuals in facilitator roles employing a range of enabling, facilitation strategies. Facilitator roles can operate at the level of novice, experienced and expert facilitators, both internally and externally to the organisational setting where implementation is taking place. Facilitation strategies focus on issues relating to the innovation, the recipients and the inner and outer context and encompass a range of technical, project management, process-related, interpersonal and influencing and negotiating skills.

The case study data present examples of the different facilitator roles, typically involving a combination of internal–external and novice–experienced–expert facilitators working together. Indeed the case studies reinforce the need for a supportive structure to be in place to mentor and guide facilitators who are new to the role. This is important given the range of issues that are encountered during a typical implementation project and the learning process that novice facilitators go through. The data suggest that a good starting point for novice facilitators is on the more direct project-related issues, for example, clarifying the project aims and goals, ascertaining the available evidence base to underpin the innovation, establishing an implementation or improvement team, undertaking a baseline assessment and developing a project outline or plan. This also has the benefit of tapping into the motivational aspects of implementation at the recipient level, as goal setting helps to create a commitment to change amongst the intended target groups for implementation. At the outset – and an important consideration in relation to facilitator recruitment and selection – essential requirements for the facilitator role include good project management skills, alongside well-developed interpersonal and communication skills and an open-minded and adaptable mind-set.

However, as already discussed, it is important not to underestimate the impact that contextual factors have on the processes and outcomes of implementation. The learning from the case studies highlights the central role that context – at the team, organisational and health system level – plays. This is a challenging issue in terms of facilitator preparation and development. Although understanding and responding to factors in the inner and outer context is essential for effective implementation, it is not an easy thing to prepare novice facilitators for, as knowledge and skills are developed and refined through experiential learning and reflection. This is where input from more experienced facilitators, who have a deeper understanding of the barriers and enablers to implementation, is invaluable. Without this mentoring and support from more experienced facilitators, novice facilitators may feel overwhelmed or ill-equipped to deal with the challenges they face. As we saw in one of the earlier chapters, this can leave the individuals in the novice facilitator role feeling isolated and exposed. In turn, this suggests a need for more structured programmes to identify, prepare and support facilitators, along the lines of the network approach encompassing novice, experienced and expert facilitators that we outlined in Chapters 5 and 7.

Issues to be explored further

This leads us to consider the things that we still do not know or where we need to further develop and test out our understanding. One interesting reflection when comparing the i-PARIHS framework to other developments in the field of evidence-based practice, knowledge translation, implementation science and innovation is the convergence of thinking. As an illustration of this, comparing the i-PARIHS framework with the Consolidated Framework for Implementation Research (CFIR), described in Chapter 3 (Damschroder et al., 2009) is interesting. Both contain similar constructs relating to the 'what, who and where' aspects of implementation (Box 13.2). The CFIR highlights the need to address the process of implementation, equivalent to the i-PARIHS concept of facilitation. Within the i-PARIHS framework, our additional focus is on how this process is activated and by whom, namely via individuals and teams working as facilitators and using facilitation strategies. Specifying these roles and the methods they can use is, we think, an important step forward in operationalising theories and frameworks of implementation.

BOX 13.2 COMPARING DOMAINS AND CONSTRUCTS IN THE i-PARIHS FRAMEWORK AND THE CONSOLIDATED FRAMEWORK FOR IMPLEMENTATION RESEARCH

Focus of implementation	The Consolidated Framework for Implementation Research	The i-PARIHS Framework
What	Intervention characteristics	Innovation
Who	Characteristics of individuals	Recipients: individual and collective
Where	Inner setting Outer setting	Context: inner local, inner organisation and outer
How	Process of implementation: planning, engaging, executing, reflecting and evaluating	Facilitator roles: novice, experienced and expert Facilitation process: clarify and engage, assess and measure, action and implementation, review and share

---

What is apparent from the current state of the science is that we seem to be coming to similar conclusions in emphasising the need for implementation approaches that embrace complexity, learning, networks, behaviour change and context. In the future, we perhaps need to be less concerned with developing more or better frameworks and focus on how we can best apply them in the real world. Or in other words, apply the principles of translational science to our own research! This calls for practitioners and researchers of implementation to work closely together developing, applying and evaluating what works, how, why and when in real-world settings. Building communities of practice amongst novice, experienced and expert facilitators is one way that we think we could move this agenda further forward. We recognise though that there is a need to check out and test the i-PARIHS framework from both a methodological and practical perspective; we will return to this in the final sections.

As already outlined, there also seems to be real potential and an opportunity to think about how to bring the concepts of evidence-based practice, knowledge translation, implementation, innovation and improvement much closer together at a clinical, organisation, policy and academic level. Fundamentally they are all working to the same aims of improving healthcare. Each has particular strengths and areas for development. For example, the innovation and improvement field has a strong history of experimentation and action, but is sometimes criticised for its lack of rigour or application of evidence. By contrast, the field of evidence-based practice and implementation science has adopted a position of systematically developing and evaluating evidence of effectiveness at a clinical, practice and organisational level. Increasingly, this has involved applying existing theories around individual and organisational behaviour change to inform the knowledge translation process; however, critics suggest that the need for prior proof considerably delays the process of innovation and change. In the words of Davidoff (2011), we have a situation of the 'evangelists and the snails' – maybe we need to give some serious thought to how we can work together across disciplines in a timely yet rigorous way to accelerate evidence-based innovation.

Where next?

In terms of the next steps, from a reader's perspective, we hope that you can use the material within the book to help plan, guide and structure your own facilitation journey, whether you are a novice in the role or trying to set up a programme of developing and supporting others to become facilitators. There is a lot of material covered in the preceding chapters and we are aware that we paint a picture of a facilitation process that is complex and wide in scope. This is because our own experience has indicated that this is the situation in most projects in most organisations. Our suggestion would be to reflect on where you are in terms of your prior knowledge and experience and concentrate of developing your understanding and skills at that level in the first instance. An appreciation of the whole process is helpful, but in terms of building expertise and confidence in the facilitator role, we would recommend applying the experiential learning methods that underpin the facilitation model, including support and mentorship from a more experienced facilitator.

For us, the next steps involve refining a set of teaching materials to accompany the i-PARIHS framework and the facilitation model that we have proposed to operationalise it. This will then enable us to set up more structured education and development programmes for facilitators and begin to build facilitation networks so that we can share learning and experiences. We also plan to undertake some further work mapping the theoretical antecedents of i-PARIHS. It is clear that 'implementation' draws on a wide range of theories at the level of individuals, teams, organisations and systems. Better understanding of these theories is one way to gain insight into which factors are important to consider in designing and researching implementation in the field. This will further guide and inform our thinking as we test out the i-PARIHS framework through both formative and summative evaluation studies. Continuing the way that we have worked with the PARIHS framework to date, we plan to use i-PARIHS and the facilitation model to design and evaluate implementation studies in real-time and to consider the development of metrics that can be used in a diagnostic, predictive and evaluative way. There are still many unknowns, including the relative importance of characteristics of the innovation, the recipients and the context and what this means in terms of the knowledge and skill requirements for facilitators. Our understanding of some of these issues will develop as ongoing programmes of research are completed and reported, such as the FIRE (Facilitating

Implementation of Research Evidence) study we have been involved in (Seers et al., 2012) and that we described in Chapter 9. Equally, new studies will be needed to drill down into outstanding questions and areas of uncertainty.

Some final thoughts

We started off writing this book because it seemed like a good idea at the time! Undertaking the background work has forced us to look more closely at a framework (PARIHS) that we developed with colleagues in a largely inductive way and which seemed to reflect others' experiences of trying to implement evidence-based practice in healthcare. This led us into examining the theoretical foundations of PARIHS, from which we came to the general conclusion that our views about implementation were firmly underpinned by concepts of individual, team and organisational learning; hence the relevance of facilitation as a means of enabling and integrating learning at these different levels. A consequence of this more detailed investigation and analysis was the integrated PARIHS (i-PARIHS) framework, a revision to the original version, which we thought was important to set out before we described an operational model of facilitation. We are now at the point where we are suggesting that facilitation is the active ingredient that integrates action around the innovation, the recipients and the context. And we have proposed a network of roles encompassing novice, experienced and expert facilitators to provide the necessary level of facilitation to initiate, implement and embed innovation in practice.

At this point in the journey, we think the i-PARIHS framework provides a good basic structure for planning, undertaking and evaluating implementation projects. The Facilitation Toolkit represents our first operational model to apply the framework in practice. We recognise there is more work to do, as the model needs to be tested, refined and further improved through repeated application and evaluation. This will form part of our ongoing journey. Essentially we are both practitioners and researchers of implementation and our interest lies in the middle ground between theory, research and practice in facilitating implementation. We hope that this book connects with your own interest and experience in evidence-based practice and innovation and provides a useful resource for implementation. We would be delighted to hear your feedback on the ideas contained within the book and suggestions for developing and improving them further (gillian.harvey@adelaide.edu.au; alison.kitson@adelaide.edu.au).

References

Damschroder, L., Aron, D., Keith, R., Kirsh, S., Alexander, J. & Lowery, J. 2009. Fostering implementation of health services research findings into practice: a consolidated framework for advancing implementation science. *Implementation Science*, 4, 50.

Davidoff, F. 2011. Systems of service: reflections on the moral foundations of improvement. *BMJ Quality & Safety*, 20, i5–i10.

Seers, K., Cox, K., Crichton, N., Edwards, R., Eldh, A., Estabrooks, C., et al. 2012. FIRE (facilitating implementation of research evidence): a study protocol. Implementation Science, 7, 25.

INDEX

Printed in the United States
by Baker & Taylor Publisher Services